THE
DIABETES
SOURCEBOOK

Today's Methods and Ways to Give Yourself the Best Care

Diana W. Guthrie, R.N., Ph.D., and
Richard A. Guthrie, M.D.

Foreword by
June Biermann and Barbara Toohey

LOWELL HOUSE
Los Angeles
CONTEMPORARY BOOKS
Chicago

Library of Congress Cataloging-in-Publication Data

Guthrie, Diana W.
   The diabetes sourcebook : today's methods and
ways to give yourself the best care / Diana W.
Guthrie and Richard A. Guthrie : foreword by
June Biermann and Barbara Toohey.
     p.   cm.
   Includes bibliographical references and index.
   ISBN 1-56565-261-4
   1. Diabetes—Popular works.   I. Guthrie,
Richard A., 1935– . II. Title.
RC660.4.G88   1992
616.4 62—dc20   92-3237
                                    CIP

     Lowell House
     2029 Century Park East, Suite 3290
     Los Angeles, CA 90067

Publisher: JACK ARTENSTEIN

General Manager, Lowell House Adult: BUD
SPERRY

Design: MIKE YAZZOLINO

Manufactured in the United States of America
10 9 8 7 6 5 4 3

This book is dedicated
to our family for the sacrifices they
made so that we would have time to write
this book, and to June Biermann and Barbara Toohey
for the tremendous contributions they have made
to people who have diabetes.

———————

Having diabetes is like learning to think
and act for the pancreas.

—DOROTHEA SIMS

Contents

Foreword

We first met Diana Guthrie back in 1979, when we were all nominated for the Ames Award as Outstanding Diabetes Educator of the Year. Diana won. As we became better acquainted with her and her endocrinologist husband, Richard, we quickly understood why. The Guthries, in their Wichita diabetes practice and their teaching at the University of Kansas Medical School at Wichita, have always been in the forefront of diabetes therapy and education and have generously given of themselves and their time to patients and colleagues.

We were often recipients of that generosity. When we wrote our *Diabetic's Total Health Book* and were advocating the then-controversial relaxation therapies for stress reduction to lower blood sugars, we were able to draw heavily on the creative and innovative work done by the Guthries, work that vividly demonstrated the benefits of these therapies for diabetics and brought them into the realm of acceptance that they enjoy today.

Whenever we write a book on diabetes or our newsletter for diabetics, the *Health-O-Gram,* we continually rely on the Guthries for advice and counsel and fact checking. They have never let us and our readers down.

To give you an idea of the measure of respect the Guthries

enjoy, once at an American Diabetes Association Annual Scientific Meeting, we were distributing complimentary copies of our *Diabetic's Total Health Book*, for which Diana had written the foreword. A large, formidable, and grouchy-looking woman, whose badge indicated that she was a diabetes nurse-educator, loomed up before our table. "What's going on here?" she demanded.

"We're giving away copies of our new book."

She picked up a copy and looked it over with a jaundiced eye.

"It's free," we chorused brightly.

She still looked skeptical. Then her eye fell on Diana's name on the cover. "Well, if Diana Guthrie had something to do with it, it must be all right. I'll take one." With that she thrust the book into her tote bag and strode off.

And then not long ago we were talking to one of the country's leading endocrinologists—a former president of the American Association of Diabetes Educators. He had just relocated his practice from South Dakota to Kansas City. When we asked him why the move, he said, "I wanted to be closer to the Source."

"The Source?"

"Yes, the Diabetes Source, you know, the Guthries in Wichita."

This book will bring you to the Source, to the Guthries and all their knowledge, experience, and empathy. Drink freely here of the waters of health and life.

June Biermann
Barbara Toohey

Introduction

Diabetes mellitus is a disease (or, more properly, a syndrome or group of diseases) that is being diagnosed with increasing frequency. The number of magazines devoted to diabetes is growing; new information is being made available to both professionals and the public as research reveals the possibilities and the problems. This book is meant to be a resource for people who have diabetes and for their family members. It is not intended to give all the answers but to serve as a guide to further reading and resources. Health-care professionals may also find this book useful as a tool for reviewing or increasing their education about the disease and its care.

When a person is diagnosed as having this syndrome, the diagnosis affects not only that person but the rest of the family as well. Information is essential, both for understanding the disease and for preventing misconceptions.

There are varying theories as to what diabetes is and how it affects the body, and there are also various approaches to treating the disease. Therefore, ongoing education should be a significant part of a treatment program. This book presents updated information on self-care and includes some of the latest research. Perhaps even more important are the suggestions for how to work with health professionals.

This book is intended not to replace classroom learning but to serve as a resource once that classroom information has been obtained. Supporting and teaching one another aids in the development of a good attitude about self-care, as does recognizing that there are many others in the same situation.

We trust that this will be a useful book. The resources found in the appendixes should aid the reader in finding out more about the various topics discussed in the chapters. We recognize that as soon as this book is printed, new information will be available that will clearly not be included in these pages. The contents of this book will, we hope, stimulate the reader to stay aware of changes and information concerning diabetes.

Many people have contributed to this book, both directly and indirectly. Our mentor, Dr. Robert Jackson, has given us the appreciation of what we as professionals can learn from those who have the disease and from their family members. Our diabetes team—Deborah Hinnen, Lindy Childs, Judy Friesen, Kirby Conley, Karon Giles, Diana Speelman, Jayne McDaniels, Mary Muncrief, Terry Burlakoff, Alicia Buckley, Marvel Logan, Julie Jamison, and Diane Mann—have contributed ideas, thoughts, or examples that were appropriate to the information presented on these pages. Their special areas of expertise have helped to make this book the resource that it is.

Special thanks go to Sharon Buller and Val Ring for their secretarial work. Special thanks go, too, to our children and grandchildren, who continually stimulate us to learn even more.

Someday, diabetes will be curable or, at least, preventable. Until then, it can be controlled. We trust that this book will aid those with the disease in controlling it, while living lives whose quality is enhanced by self-care practices.

Chapter 1

What Kind of Diabetes Do You Have?

Diabetes is not a single disease with a single cause. Rather, it is a collection of diseases, some more difficult to control than others. All forms of diabetes involve a hormone (body regulator) from the pancreas called insulin. If you have diabetes, either you lack insulin or the insulin you have is not doing its job properly. The result is that instead of being stored for energy through the action of insulin, the foods you eat (primarily the starches or carbohydrates) raise your blood sugar to higher-than-normal levels. Without treatment, your blood sugar remains high and has the potential of adversely affecting every organ and system in your body. With treatment, the insulin problem can be solved, and your blood sugar can be brought down or normalized so that the body is not damaged. A person with diabetes can thus remain healthy and look forward to a normal life span.

A Bit of History

An ancient Egyptian papyrus described diabetes as a disease that caused a person to "melt into the loins." The name itself indicates the loss of valuable body fluids: diabetes is from a

Greek word, meaning to siphon. *Mellitus,* a Roman word, relates to a word meaning "sweet tasting." Yes, due to the high sugar content and the lack of earlier testing methodologies, actually tasting the urine did give an indication that the person had "sugar diabetes"! In fact, Mother Nature was fooling the disease's early observers, who saw the crystalline content of the urine after its liquid contents had evaporated. In the fourteenth century, this was actually thought to be a salt (people were not into taste-testing at that time, we suppose).

Diabetes mellitus was treated, over time, by various means aimed at lowering the sugar content in the urine or decreasing the loss of fluid. Some patients fasted and feasted on alternating days, weeks, or months. Others were taught to eat rancid meat or vegetables cooked "three times in their own water." Others survived on eggs or cereal. The association of food and fluid was passed down through time. Eventually, the discovery was made that the hormone insulin, secreted by cells called the islets of Langerhans, needed to be replaced in the body in order for normal blood-glucose levels to be achieved.

Many people contributed to the knowledge about monitoring blood-glucose levels. Insulin could not be analyzed or its significant contact noted until the 1960s. We learned that other hormones, such as glucagon, might help cause the disease. We also learned that diabetes is not the result of a single event in the body but of several events that lead to a series of immune responses, with the end result being that the majority of insulin-making cells (beta cells, found in the islets of Langerhans) are no longer working.

With the discovery of insulin, many people believed that diabetes had been cured. However, it was found that if the person lived longer than the expected two or so years, and especially if the blood-glucose levels were not significantly controlled for the majority of the time, complications occurred (for example, blindness, heart disease, or the need for amputation). Many of these complications can now be prevented or delayed with proper medical care. For example, vision problems can now be stabilized. Amputations, the complication most associated with diabetes in its earlier days, can be prevented in an increasing number of cases. In addition, problems that can occur with certain organs (e.g., heart, kidneys, or liver) can be reversed or treated with transplantation, something unheard of in the first half of this century.

Education of the diabetes patient is one of the major keys to attaining such high degrees of control. Since health professionals cannot be with the person and his or her family on a day-in, day-out basis, self-management education is a must.

Types of Diabetes

Diabetes has been divided into three groups: Type I, or insulin-dependent diabetes mellitus (IDDM), in which insulin must be injected daily; Type II, or non–insulin dependent diabetes mellitus (NIDDM), in which insulin injection is usually not necessary; and secondary diabetes (due to pancreatic surgery or over-active glands, such as the pituitary or the adrenals). We are concerned here only with Type I and Type II diabetes.

Type I diabetes is believed to be caused by a combination of genetics and environmental stressors. The individual who becomes Type I develops an inability to make insulin. When insulin is absent, the cells are in a state of starvation, while an excess of sugar—in the form of glucose—is made available in the blood. This state of high blood glucose is called *hyperglycemia* or, in this case, diabetes mellitus. (Hyperglycemia may be caused by a number of stressors, but when it is due to problems with insulin it is called diabetes mellitus.) Despite eating vast amounts of food, the person remains in a condition of starvation until adequate insulin is available and can get the food into the cells. Body fat is burned as an alternate fuel; a by-product, *ketone bodies*, are created as a source of energy. But ketones cause the accumulation of acids and upset the body's buffer system. The body develops a serious problem known as *ketoacidosis*, a chemical imbalance of the body accompanied by high blood sugar. This creates the classic symptoms of out-of-control diabetes: frequent urination (polyuria), excessive thirst (polydipsia), and excessive hunger (polyphagia). If neglected, ketoacidosis can eventually lead to death.

Type II diabetes, besides being called non–insulin dependent diabetes, has also been known by many other names, such as maturity onset diabetes, non–ketosis prone, ketosis resistant, and even MODY, for "maturity onset diabetes in the young." Eighty to 85 percent of the diabetic population is diagnosed as having Type II diabetes. Of these, 88 percent or so are overweight. Many of the so-called "borderline diabetics" are Type IIs.

Insulin is still the key factor in this disease, but often there is an excess of it rather than a lack. The increase in insulin is believed to be the result of overeating. The excess insulin causes a decrease in the cell's number of insulin-receptor sites (that is, links to get the insulin into the cell). In the absence of receptor sites, the insulin does not work, and the result is diabetes (hyperglycemia). While the elevation in blood-glucose levels may lead to polyuria, polydipsia, and polyphagia, as in Type I diabetes, a key difference exists.

In the majority of Type IIs there is a history of weight gain rather than weight loss as happens in out-of-control Type I. This is caused by a sort of a "chicken or egg" phenomenon: the excess insulin increases appetite and results in increased food intake. The excess food that causes the excess insulin in the blood and the loss of insulin receptors also causes the weight gain characteristic of Type II diabetes. The weight gain is particularly understandable in light of insulin's major purpose: storage.

Type II diabetes is most often diagnosed in individuals over 30 years old and is relatively slow in onset. The diminished and/or faulty insulin-site receptors lead to what physicians normally call "insulin resistance." This is the term frequently used to explain to Type II patients what the difference is between their diabetes and Type I, which involves "insulin lack."

Both types can be either insulin-requiring or non–insulin requiring, and both can experience a decrease in their insulin-making ability to the point where they become insulin-dependent. At times it is difficult to state whether an individual is really a Type I (insulin-dependent diabetes mellitus, or IDDM) or Type II (non–insulin dependent diabetes mellitus, or NIDDM). A laboratory test that gives an indication of how much insulin, if any, a person is secreting can be used to differentiate the two types.

Problems Associated with Diabetes

With Type I (insulin-dependent) diabetes, after the acute episode (diabetic ketoacidosis) or early symptoms leading to the diagnosis (frequent passing of urine, normal eating with weight loss, extreme thirst), there may be a partial remission period (the "honeymoon") in which the body appears to be able to make some insulin again. This period usually lasts from three to six months, but it may last longer, depending on the suppression of the insulin-making ability of the beta cells through an external insulin-injection program. Illness or extreme emotional stress appear to aid in further destruction of the beta cells, as does growth, and may shorten the remission period. Eventually, the person becomes totally insulin dependent, especially if more than 90 percent of the beta cells become inactive.

Type II diabetes is a serious disease. Insulin-resistant, non–ketosis prone people most often have elevated insulin levels, which aids in the process that leads to obesity (since the basic function of insulin is storage). The large amounts of insulin in the Type II person might be due to insulin resistance (loss of ability to use insulin correctly), increased hepatic (liver) glucose making, or problems with post-receptor (inside the cell) function. Since even one dose of insulin results in the development of antibodies, oral glucose-tolerance tests (the taking of a blood sample, giving a drink high in sugar, and repeated taking of blood samples—for example, every half-hour for two hours, or longer) done at that time would not be exact. Measurement of C-peptide gives more information as to whether a person is secreting insulin or not, because it measures internal, or endogenous, insulin secretion. C-peptide is the third link in the chain that "breaks off," leaving the two-chain insulin chemical. The chains are made up of a series of specific amino acids (protein) in a specific order. C-peptide eventually finds its way into the bloodstream, as does insulin, but is considered only a waste product.

Except during the "honeymoon," or partial-remission, period, persons with IDDM do not have the ability to secrete C-peptide. Persons with NIDDM usually can secrete adequate, or even elevated, amounts of C-peptide. Even patients with NIDDM often become insulin dependent with time as the pancreas becomes exhausted from the extra secretion of insulin.

Chapter 2

Who Gets This Disease?

In 1977, the Diabetes Data Group (a government-appointed group of the National Diabetes Advisory Board) reported that an estimated $6 billion is spent each year in this country on diabetes, for direct costs (medical care) and indirect costs (lost work time, etc.). In 1984, according to the report, "Diabetes in America," the loss was reportedly $14 billion annually. And in 1989, the cost was estimated to be $20.6 billion—roughly 3.6 percent of total U.S. health-care costs. This is an average cost per year of $2,000 for each insulin-dependent person. Many studies have been reported that show great cost savings— as much as $3 million per year, in one program (Miller, 1982)—through patient teaching and proper medical care.

Early Forms of Diabetes

Once called chemical diabetes or prediabetes, early forms of carbohydrate intolerance include impaired glucose tolerance, previous abnormality of glucose tolerance, and potential abnormality of glucose tolerance. Impaired glucose tolerance is the diagnosis of a person with a normal fasting sugar (glucose) level who, after drinking a certain amount of a liquid that contains sugar (glucose), has one value above 200 mg/dl, or 11 mMol. The measurement "mMol" is metric. To convert mg/dl to mMol for blood sugar, divide by 18. For example: 200 mg/dl ÷ 18 = 11 mMol.

Insulin values may be low-normal, high-normal, or, in many cases, have a delay in release. The delayed release may then lead to an excess release of insulin. The result of the delayed insulin release is a drop in blood sugar, called reactive hypoglycemia. Previous abnormality of glucose tolerance means that at a time in the past the person experienced hyperglycemia—perhaps associated with a heart attack, a severe burn, or other highly stressful situation (such as pregnancy)—but now has a normal glucose-tolerance test. Potential abnormality of glucose tolerance describes high-risk individuals—for example, those who are overweight; women with a history of multiple stillbirths, miscarriages, or babies weighing more than nine pounds at birth; or individuals with a strong family history of the disease.

Gestational Diabetes

Gestational diabetes develops during pregnancy and may revert back to impaired glucose tolerance or previous abnormality of glucose tolerance after the pregnancy is over. It is possible that this individual will progress to diabetes of either Type I (IDDM) or Type II (NIDDM). Further testing is needed if the fasting blood-sugar level is above 105 mg/dl (5.8 or 6 mMol), or if a two-hour postmeal (postprandial) blood-sugar level is greater than 150 mg/dl (8 mMol).

The present recommendation is that not only should high-risk pregnant females be screened, but all pregnant females should be screened by the twenty-fourth to twenty-eighth week of gestation. Statistics show that prepregnancy control of blood-sugar (glucose) levels among pregnant diabetic women leads to mother and infant outcomes that are nearly the same as for non-diabetic pregnant women. If control is achieved only by the time of the second trimester, there is a 14 percent chance that the infant will die or develop complications, such as heart, head, or spinal malformations. The mother will have more problems with toxemia and eclampsia. The second trimester is the time in which the stresses of pregnancy begin to show, and these effects elevate the blood-sugar levels. Treatment should begin promptly and continue from early in the pregnancy to the end.

Secondary Types of Diabetes

Secondary types of diabetes are due to a number of causes or states, such as injury to or surgical removal of the pancreas. Additional causes are associated with inflammation of the pancreas (pancreatitis) or elevated plasma iron associated with an enlarged liver, pigmentation of the skin, and (frequently) cardiac failure. Hormonal diseases such as Cushing's disease (puffy red face) or acromegaly (large face, long arms and hands) may also cause diabetes.

Causes of Diabetes

Drugs such as steroids, Dilantin, and others may elevate the blood sugar through a variety of mechanisms. Certain other drugs, such as alloxan, streptozocin, and thiazide diuretics, are toxic to the beta cells of the pancreas and can cause diabetes. Certain syndromes (for example, Prader-Willi, Down's, progeria, and Turner's) may result in a hyperglycemic state; if this state is prolonged, the result can be permanent (that is, insulin-dependent) diabetes.

Diabetes resulting in an insulin-dependent state is classified as Type I diabetes. While Type I diabetes affects only between 10 and 15 percent of the diabetic population, its effects on the body can be worse than other forms of diabetes. In the past, Type I has been known as juvenile or juvenile-onset diabetes (because it is usually diagnosed in those under thirty), brittle diabetes, unstable diabetes, and ketosis-prone diabetes. People in this classification more frequently exhibit the classic symptoms. A fasting blood-sugar level of 140 mg/dl (8 mMol) or above and two or more other blood-sugar levels over 200 mg/dl (11 mMol), usually with ketones present in blood and urine, indicate the presence of Type I diabetes. A blood-sugar level of 800 mg/dl (44 mMol) or more, especially if ketones are not present, indicates a diagnosis of hyperglycemic hyperosmolar nonketotic syndrome (a state in which the body is extremely dry [dehydrated], the chemicals in the body are concentrated, and the blood sugar is high).

As stated before, diabetes is a syndrome, or group of diseases (rather than one disease), leading to the prolonged hyperglycemic state. Type I is most associated with the killing of the beta cells, most likely by the body's own immune system. Either the immune system cannot kill an infecting agent, which then kills the beta cells, or the immune system itself goes "wild," attacking the body's own tissue and destroying the beta cells. The cells of the islets of Langerhans are inflamed, resulting from an infectious-disease process (for example, mumps) or, more commonly, from an autoimmune (allergic to self) response.

The autoimmune process results in the circulation of antibodies that may either cause or be caused by beta-cell death. If it is found that the antibodies cause beta-cell destruction (the body fighting what it now considers foreign to itself), the body's response to the Type I diabetes is much less severe (i.e., easier to control) with treatment. Until then, the outcome is a lack of available insulin. While the onset is said to be sudden, changes resulting in decreased insulin availability may have occurred over a longer period of time. In short, insulin-dependent diabetes mellitus (IDDM) is an inherited defect of the body's immune system, resulting in destruction of the insulin-producing beta cells of the pancreas.

Heredity is a major cause of diabetes. If both parents have Type II diabetes, there is a chance that nearly all of their children will have diabetes. If both parents have Type I diabetes, fewer than 20 percent of their children will develop Type I diabetes. In identical twins, if one twin develops Type II diabetes, the chance is nearly 100 percent that the other twin will also develop it. In Type I diabetes, however, only 40 to 50 percent of the second twins will develop the disease, indicating that while inheritance is important, environmental factors (for example, too much food, too much stress, viral infection, and so forth) are also involved in the development of Type I diabetes.

Causes of Type I Diabetes

Type I Diabetes is an inherited defect of the immune system triggered by an environmental stimuli. The problem may be in the on switch of the immune system in which the viral stimuli does not turn the system on. The virus then is allowed to penetrate the beta cell and cause its destruction. Conversely, the problem may be in the off switch in that the system turns on appropriately and kills the virus but then does not turn itself off. The T-Killer cells are then allowed to attack the beta cells themselves. This is a very simplified explanation. In point of fact, it is much more complex, involving many, many steps in the immune system. The beta cells themselves may contribute to this by producing antigens or chemicals on the cell surface which stimulate the immune system and there may be many other environmental stimuli rather than just viruses. Indeed there is some evidence now that proteins in cows milk may cause the formation of antibodies which can attach to the beta cell or which are similar to antibodies on the beta cell. When the immune system mobilizes in response to a stimulus, these antibodies will attach to receptors on the cell surface of the beta cell causing the damage to occur to the beta cells of the pancreas. For whatever reason, the beta cells are then destroyed by the immune system in what is called an auto-immune phenomena, in which the body has come to recognize itself as a foreign body and begins to eliminate certain parts.

Recently researchers have been attempting to locate the genes for diabetes. As a part of the genome project, in which researchers around the world are attempting to map the entire gene structure of all of the human chromosomes, they have isolated 18 genes which appear to be involved in the production of type I diabetes. Not all these genes have equal potency. Two of them appear to be most potent, as some others are least potent and others are simply auxiliary or helper genes that seem to have some assisting effect in the process. There are also genes which are protective so that one might inherit the genes for diabetes but if you also inherited the protective genes, you would not develop the disease. Thus development of the disease is not 100% in those who have inherited the genetics for the disease. Those people may have the genes but they may either have protector genes or they may be fortunate enough to avoid the environmental stimuli.

Summary

The cause of Type I diabetes, then, is an inherited defect in the immune system which interacts in some way with environmental factors. These factors may be viruses or chemicals in the environment or perhaps other environmental factors, that we have not yet identified, which team up together to result in the eventual complete destruction of the beta cells and the loss of insulin secretion.

Type II Diabetes

The cause of type II diabetes is not as well understood. Two factors appear to be important in type II diabetes. These are insulin resistance and insulin deficiency. There is a debate over which comes first but the general consensus of the moment is that insulin resistance is the first factor. Type II diabetes is also a genetic disease although the genes are carried on entirely different chromosomes than those for Type I diabetes. There are probably multiple genes involved in this disease. For whatever reason, this genetic factor perhaps interacting with some environmental factors such as overweight, excess caloric intake, deficient caloric expenditure, and aging may result then in a resistance to insulin. That is the peripheral cell, a muscle or fat or other cell, does not respond appropriately to the insulin which is present. The body then begins to produce more insulin in order to try to overcome the insulin resistance. The next part of the sequence may involve two factors. One is the increasing insulin secretion may ultimately exhaust the beta cells resulting in insulin deficiency. Another factor has recently been indentified and this is called glucotoxicity or sugar toxicity. It turns out that sugar in high amounts can be toxic or poisonous to the cells of the body. In the person with insulin resistance who is running high blood sugars that have been undetected and untreated or even in the person with the disease who knows it and who does not treat it appropriately, the continuing high levels of sugar have a toxic effect on the insulin producing cells of the pancreas damaging those cells and reducing insulin secretion. So we then end up with a combination of peripheral resistance to the action of insulin and at the same time insulin deficiency and those two then can precipitate a severe case of type II diabetes which may in fact require insulin for treatment. There are many steps in the action of insulin at the peripheral cell level and each of those steps is stimulated by a different enzyme and each enzyme is controlled by a different gene, therefore, there are many potential places where the defects can occur resulting in the same ultimate end which is resistance of the peripheral cell to the action of insulin which is probably the precipitating factor in type II diabetes.

There is an increase in the diabetes for both Type I and Type II disease but a more pronounced increase in Type II. The increase is at the rate of about 6% per year which means the number of people with diabetes will double every fifteen years. In the US this increase is occurring predominately in the non-white ethnic populations. The prevalence of diabetes in the caucasian population is approximately 5–6% in the black population is somewhere between 12–15%. In the hispanic population it is around 20% and in the native american population they frequently exceed 30%. Indeed there are tribes in which the prevalence may be as much as 65%. Likewise diabetes is increasing in the world particularly in developing countries. The disease is very rare in third world or undeveloped countries. But as those countries begin to develop and achieve industrial prominence and economic stability is a mushrooming of the amount of diabetes in those cultures. This was seen in Japan after World War II and most recently in Korea and Taiwan and is now occurring in other southeast Asian countries as the standard of living begins to increase. It is thought that this increase is probably related to increased caloric intake associated with decreased caloric expenditure. The genes for type II diabetes are probably widespread throughout the world of equal amount in all races and ethnic groups but the change in lifestyle from manual labor with a low caloric intake to industrial labor with a high caloric intake and reduced caloric expenditure, because of the use of machinery, can then result in a virtual explosion of Type II.

Type I diabetes also has a difference in geographic areas. The difference appears not to be so much between racial or ethnic groups but that of geography. It is lowest near the equator and as one moves farther north to the arctic circle the prevalence of the disease increases. The highest prevalence being in the Scandinavian countries. The lowest in the mediterranean area except for the Island of Sardinia which has an incidence equal to that of Finland. The reasons for these differences are not well understood and are currently the source of investigation.

Chapter 3

How Is Diabetes Treated?

The treatment of diabetes mellitus must be varied from person to person and from time to time. The goals are listed in Table 3-1.

A variety of things affect the treatment of this disease for each individual. There are, for one thing, personal changes (for example, changing jobs, moving, and taking on new responsibilities). There is a change in response from morning to

TABLE 3-1

IDEAL VS. ACCEPTABLE BLOOD SUGARS

BLOOD-SUGAR GOALS	IDEAL	ACCEPTABLE
Fasting blood sugar	70–110 mg/dl (4–6 mMol)	60–120 mg/dl (3–7 mMol)
1 hour after meal	90–150 mg/dl (5–8 mMol)	80–180 mg/dl (4–10 mMol)
2 hours after meal	84–140 mg/dl (5–8 mMol)	70–150 mg/dl (4–8 mMol)
3 hours after meal	60–100 mg/dl (3–6 mMol)	60–130 mg/dl (3–7 mMol)

Average blood sugars for a pregnant woman with diabetes should be around 90 mg/dl (5 mMol).

---

afternoon, and from noon to midnight. If a person is highly stressed, there is going to be a difference. If the person is relaxed, there is going to be a difference. The type of diabetes will also make a difference. (Note that a person who does not have diabetes will have very little change in blood sugar even after eating a whole box of candy, but the person with diabetes will have an elevated blood sugar.) The following sections describe some of these differences and tell you how you can share this information with your health professional.

Differences in Treatment for Children and Adults

A child cannot be treated as a miniature adult. A one-unit change in insulin in a 40-pound child will have much more of an effect than a one-unit change in a 140-pound adult. Children have not only rapidly changing size but also rapidly changing hormones. These changing hormones lead to various changes in emotional responses. In some children with Type I diabetes, the disease is more severe; if beta-cell function is preserved, it may be more mild. More food is needed for a child's active lifestyle as well as for growth and development.

As with any type of diabetes, the goal is to attain and maintain a high degree of control of blood-glucose levels and a quality of life that makes it all worthwhile. If a child does not get enough to eat and enough insulin to help get food into the cells for energy and growth, he or she will not grow at all or will not grow at the rate expected.

If blood sugars are normalized most of the time, the only time a child should ever become ill with diabetes is at diagnosis, when diabetic ketoacidosis (high blood-glucose levels, dehydration, and chemical [electrolyte] imbalance) is present. Learning when it is possible to have a higher blood sugar and to give more insulin before the body gets out of control prevents diabetic keto-acidosis from ever occurring again. Often, diabetic ketoacidosis can be predicted (for example, if there is an infection). More fluids and more insulin, as needed, would keep this problem from occurring. Checking for ketones in the urine would tell the parents whether the body is using fats for an energy source. If the blood-glucose levels are high (300 mg/dl [17 mMol] or greater), the body can become chemically out of balance and the child can become very sick.

Low blood-glucose levels (hypoglycemia) are the other side of the coin. This is a little more difficult to handle. Some people are more afraid of the short-term effects of low blood sugar than the long-term effects of high blood sugar. Some of these times can be predicted—for example, if the child is anticipating something special the next day and so is not sleeping well. If they can be predicted, then in most cases they can be prevented. If they are not predicted, rapid and early treatment is most helpful. If the symptoms or feelings are ignored or are not noticeable enough, a problem could occur.

Blood-glucose testing has been a great help in the early finding of low blood sugar. Small children may not have the words to say that they are "feeling funny." Or they might be so involved in play that they do not notice that their lowering blood sugars are giving them signals that it's time to get something to eat. If they feel hunger, there is more of a chance that they will respond by getting something to eat, but this is not always so.

A mild insulin reaction (hypoglycemia) now and then is nothing compared to frequent times of very low blood glucose. The brain can take only so much, such as the lack of a fuel source, before it will undergo cell damage. This is especially true if the reactions are of the severe type (jerking or unconsciousness). *Severe reactions must be prevented at all costs.* Mild episodes of shaking and sweating every so often, although somewhat uncomfortable to experience, are not as serious as the severe reactions. If the child has not reached the age of full nerve development (six to eight years of age), there is a greater chance that hypoglycemia will result in brain damage.

Allowing anyone—child or adult—to have high blood sugar (hyperglycemia) all the time is also not recommended. The person will be dull, less alert, and often more irritable. Teachers and employers will usually report a change in learning or working ability when the blood sugar is either too high or too low. True, the child or adult is not having insulin reactions, but in the long-term picture, a slight insulin reaction now and then is much less damaging than chronic high blood-glucose levels. Interestingly, if the blood-glucose control is poor, there is often a greater chance of having severe insulin reactions.

The chance of having more severe insulin reactions with higher blood-glucose content has been debated. The Diabetes Control and Complications Trial, a ten-year study to determine what level of control very early on will best prevent or delay complications, stated that the more normal the glucose control, the greater the chance of having severe insulin reactions. In the third year of the study, the intensive control group experienced a 30 to 40 percent increase in low blood-glucose levels compared to the standard control group. Most of the first group's hypoglycemia was without symptoms, with blood-glucose values in the forties. A year later, at the National Meeting of the American Diabetes Association it was announced that there had been a change in treatment methods and hypoglycemia had decreased dramatically. As a side comment, the speaker said he guessed they were learning how to manage diabetes better because there were fewer low blood-glucose reactions in the intensive control group. Our own experience has been that the number of severe hypoglycemic episodes is fewer, or certainly no greater, among children or adults in "tighter" control than among those with wildly swinging or chronically high blood sugars.

As diabetic ketoacidosis is usually associated with infection or prolonged emotional stress, so hypoglycemia is associated with a mistake in the amount of insulin given, a lot of play or exercise without extra food, or manipulation with food (for example, a child's refusal to eat food in order to get his or her way). This is why parent education and the type of treatment program chosen are so helpful.

Part of the parents' education includes the following: The total daily dose of insulin divided into multiple doses per day spreads out the impact of the peak, or top, action of the insulin. If you give all the insulin in one dose, it won't cover the entire twenty-four-hour time period; in addition, the strongest action time of the insulin might cause the child to be hypoglycemic then and yet hyperglycemic before the next dose is given. Spreading the doses out allows no great impact at any one time. Multiple doses doesn't mean that the diabetes is getting worse. It's just a method of allowing more flexibility in a child's lifestyle.

Psychological adjustment to the disease can develop when more flexibility is present. Children who have parents who support them often just take their diabetes in stride. Too, the younger child frequently adjusts more easily than the teenager or the adult. Parents, on the other hand, may either become too protective or may, either subconsciously or openly, reject the child. If the parents are not educated and supported by health-care professionals, the child may become upset to the point at which the diabetes becomes very hard to manage. Discipline becomes a very important part in the treatment program for the child. The more lovingly the child is disciplined, the greater the chance that he or she will have a long and healthy life.

When a group of children with diabetes was compared to a group of children who didn't, it was found that there was no greater number of conflicts or psychological diagnoses in one group than in the other. It was also noted that the diabetes management was in poorer control in the families that did not work as a team.

Acute Care

The initial management of Type I diabetes is about the same for adults and children. Most physicians will give small amounts of insulin continuously or hourly in relation to the person's size and in relation to the state of ketoacidosis and dehydration. In fact, some intravenous fluids are usually given before insulin. Just think about this: if you have a glass half filled with water and you put ten teaspoons of sugar in it, would you have a faster response in lowering the amount of sugar in each teaspoon of liquid if you put in something to use up the sugar or if you filled the glass to the top with water? It's the same with the human body. Fluid is added, then insulin is started. When the laboratory work comes back, other chemicals such as potassium are added if necessary. Also, in most cases the doctor will not add the potassium until the person passes urine (otherwise, the potassium would become too concentrated in the body and cause problems).

The rate of fall of the blood-glucose levels is usually controlled so that it does not exceed much more than 100 mg/dl (5–6 mMol) per hour. This helps the body in its rebalancing process. It also helps prevent headaches, since the brain would otherwise get too much of a jolt in having the sudden greater amount of fluid and lesser amount of sugar. Saline, or salt water, may be used first, as it aids the tissues in accepting the fluid that is needed. Later on, glucose is added to the saline, or the total intravenous fluid is changed to a glucose solution. This may seem strange when the problem was initially caused by too much glucose in the system. However, the glucose in the water does a number of things. For one, it prevents the person from becoming hypoglycemic. For another, it prevents the person from making ketones from free fatty acids when the body recognizes it needs something for energy.

To monitor the other chemicals in the body to be sure they are not out of balance, it is necessary to do blood tests every few hours. Usually, the blood is drawn through a plastic needle placed in a vein; very small amounts of heparin are put into the needle once the blood has been removed to prevent clotting (this is called a "heparin lock"). Each time a specimen is needed, the heparin fluid is withdrawn, and the amount of blood needed is removed. Heparin is then replaced into the needle space until the next specimen is needed. This step prevents the need to stick a person many times to obtain these blood specimens. This plastic needle may be kept in place until the IV is discontinued or after the first day or two (i.e., six to forty-eight hours).

Another way of testing how well a person is doing is by looking at the cardiac monitor. Not only can the nurses and doctors tell whether chemicals such as potassium are at low or high levels, they can also tell whether calcium, magnesium, or other chemicals called electrolytes are out of balance. Actually, when there is adequate fluid replacement in the face of the appropriate amount of insulin, the other chemicals seem to balance out.

Management of Type I Diabetes

Depending on the management program you are in, once the acute state of the diabetes management is controlled you may be discharged from the hospital and asked to return to the doctor on a daily, weekly, or monthly basis, plus receive some education on initial survival skills (how to administer the insulin, how to plan a meal, how to treat a reaction, how to monitor blood-glucose levels and urine ketones, and when and what to tell the doctor). You may be asked to return a few weeks or months later for more intensive education. If your stay in the hospital lasts one to two weeks or so, you will receive education and psychological support during this time.

If the hospitalization time is short, the physician will start the total amount of daily insulin delivery at a lower level and increase the dosage until the suitable level of diabetes control is achieved. With the longer hospitalization, the physician will administer what is termed a "physiological amount of insulin," based on the patient's body size and food intake. The insulin is then lowered on a daily basis until the baseline, or normal, blood-glucose levels are stabilized.

Each method has its pros and cons. The former gives less early support, allowing the person to develop habits that might not be appropriate. But it does get the person back to work or school sooner and into a scheduled lifestyle from which individual needs can be assessed. The latter approach gives more initial psychological and physiological support. With this approach, most programs try to have the person's daily lifestyle mimicked by the activity and education program planned. This approach also appears to have a longer "honeymoon" period, during which the control of blood sugar may be easily obtained through the use of small amounts of insulin. This is due to the beta cells having recovered some ability to produce insulin internally. It has not been proved that this is better in the long run, but certainly the diabetes is easier to control for a longer period of time (from six months to three or four years).

Whatever the program, it needs to be individualized, with the person's lifestyle taken into account: When are the physical education classes? When are the coffee breaks? What time is bedtime? When are meals usually eaten?—and so forth. The food should be patterned to meet the everyday needs. The insulin is then patterned to get the products of the food (such as glucose or proteins, and, indirectly, fats) to go to the places they are supposed to go. As needs and age requirements change, the program must also change. If a person becomes more sedentary, the food intake needs to be decreased and the insulin (or oral agent, for adults) decreased. If too much insulin is given, the person could either have trouble with insulin reactions or eat to compensate for the symptoms of hunger with the low blood sugar and thus become fat. As a child grows and requires more food (not just more carbohydrates, but more total calories), he or she will require more insulin. As the child becomes an adult, stops growing, and requires less food, less insulin will be required.

In the normal nondiabetic person, the body produces a small

amount of insulin continuously. This is called *basal insulin*. The body then produces a burst of insulin after each intake of food. It is this pattern that must be duplicated for the diabetic, whatever treatment regimen is chosen. For people with insulin-dependent diabetes mellitus (IDDM), this pattern can be duplicated in many ways, with many food patterns and insulin patterns (four, three, or two doses of insulin per day). The minimum requirement for duplicating the normal pattern is three meals, with one to three between-meal and bedtime snacks and an insulin pattern of two doses per day (before breakfast or supper) of a mixture of a short-acting (Regular) insulin and intermediate-acting insulin (NPH or Lente). (NPH or Lente insulins last twice as long as the short-acting insulin, or roughly half as long as the long-acting insulins.) The two doses of intermediate-acting insulin supply the twenty-four-hour basal and the coverage for lunch. The two doses of short-acting insulin provide the bursts for breakfast and supper. Usually, twice as much insulin is given in the A.M. as in the P.M., because two meals are eaten for the A.M. dose and one meal for the P.M. dose. And twice as much intermediate as short-acting insulin is usually given in each dose, since the intermediate insulin must last twelve hours, while the short-acting insulin lasts only six hours.

Management of Type II Diabetes

For some adults with mild elevations of blood sugar, redistribution of calories throughout the day (just as insulin dosages are distributed throughout the day) keeps the body from being challenged at any one time of day or may smooth out the blood-sugar levels. If weight loss or choices of food do not aid the person in maintaining an average blood sugar below 150 mg/dl (8 mMol), then the person will need some oral hypoglycemic agent to assist the body in functioning more appropriately. If an illness occurs in which a person cannot keep food down or the beta cells decrease their functioning, the person might temporarily need to go on insulin. Often, the oral agents will no longer work after five to ten years (this is called secondary failure of oral hypoglycemic agents), and the person will need to start using insulin. Especially if it is determined that the person is insulin resistant and thus actually requires high doses of insulin, some physicians find that they need to combine dosages of insulin with an oral agent given once or twice a day (see chapter 6 for more information).

Exercise becomes a very important part of the adult's management program. While children usually have planned exercise in school, the adult must exercise on his or her own. Exercise offers many benefits, one of which is a greater sensitivity to insulin by the receptor sites of the cells.

As the adult ages, the management program changes again. And if a complication of diabetes develops, many changes occur. If the problem involves the eyes, treatment will be needed to stabilize them. Adjusting to this treatment will likely cause changes in the person's activity pattern; emotions will thus be involved. If the problem involves the kidneys, blood pressure will need to be controlled. The use of medication to treat blood pressure may alter blood-glucose levels. If kidneys are affected by the aging process or by disease, the body will retain the insulin or oral-agent chemicals longer than is desired. There may thus be a need for lower doses of insulin or less of an oral agent, or a change from an oral agent to insulin.

As adults adjust to having diabetes and learn more about their own care, their diabetes control can truly be fine-tuned. The word *diabetes* does not need to be in neon lights all the time! Changes of life may seem like obstacles to the diabetic, but a better way to see them is as challenges that happen to accompany the diagnosis of diabetes.

Special Management Needs

Pregnancy

For the pregnant woman with Type I, Type II, or gestational diabetes, there are certain changes in the body's needs. Pregnancy has been called a "diabetogenic state." Pregnancy is stressful to the body, and anything that is stressful to the body results in the release of hormones that allow or cause the blood sugar to become elevated. It is a state of greater stress for the body. The metabolic rate is higher, so the body burns food faster. Greater amounts of food are needed throughout the pregnancy. As greater amounts of food are needed, more insulin is needed. Hormones produced by the placenta also increase insulin needs. On delivery, the hormones that have resulted in greater body stress stop being released. Less insulin is then needed. Breast-feeding will further reduce the insulin need. If the person has diabetes just during pregnancy, it is possible that the blood-glucose levels will return to normal four to six weeks after delivery.

Although diabetes may be detected during a routine screening sometime during the twenty-fourth to twenty-eighth week of gestation, the pregnant woman may come to the doctor's office because she is feeling unusually tired—the result of high blood sugar. High blood sugar also results in blurry vision, sores that don't heal, and frequency of urination. Symptoms like those of the flu or appendicitis may be felt. Treatment to return the blood-glucose levels to normal makes these symptoms go away. During pregnancy, it is a must to keep blood sugars normal to prevent problems for both mother and baby (see chapter 10 for more information).

Travel

Your health professional can also prepare you for travel. Another resource is the International Travel Association. You may call the National Diabetes Association and get the number of a place in New York that will tell you the names and addresses of physicians in almost any part of the world. You can also find out what equipment is available in various countries in case you run out (but try not to!). You should be able to say "I need a doctor" in the appropriate language. Traveling on planes and trains can be made much easier when you know what to eat, when to eat it, whom to contact if special meals are desired. (Again, see chapter 10 for more information.)

June Biermann and Barbara Toohey, initial developers of the SugarFree Centers, are two people who have looked at life's obstacles as challenges. June has insulin-dependent diabetes, but this has never kept her from skiing the biggest mountain or exploring the farthest island. She has done this through self-management. Learning self-management means learning how your body responds to certain amounts of food, certain kinds of food, and certain amounts of diabetes medication. It also means knowing that if you have to take other medication for colds, flu, or other health problems, you plan for this with your health professional before you travel.

Chapter 4

Educating Yourself About Diabetes

The more we learn about diabetes mellitus, the more complex it seems to become. Basic information is available that can assist the person who has diabetes to make this complex disease more simple. This information can be presented on three levels: a survival level, with just enough information to help the person (or family) in the completion of daily tasks; a home-management level, which includes the basics on almost all topics related to the disease; and a self-management level, which includes what you need to know for true self-management. Self-management involves decision making within a program that has been developed specifically for you by your physician.

Levels of Education

Basic "Survival" Level

The survival level of education includes what medication to take, how much of it to take, and when to take it. If you are giving yourself your own injections, you would be taught how to get the insulin into the syringe, how to administer the injection, and how to take care of your supplies and equipment. A meal plan would be developed, and you would be told the lists of food choices, the amounts to eat, and when they should be eaten. To keep track of yourself and to determine if what you are doing is correct, you would monitor your blood-glucose levels using a finger-stick test. If your blood-glucose levels were 250 mg/dl (14 mMol) or greater, you would be told to check your urine for ketones, especially if you were ill or taking insulin. Since below-normal blood-glucose levels might be a side effect of the administration of either oral hypoglycemic agents or insulin, you would be taught how to recognize low blood sugar and how to treat it. Most important of all, you would be taught when to contact your health professionals and what to tell them.

These are the basics, and they should be included as part of your management program before you leave the hospital or in conjunction with your initial visits to the doctor concerning diabetes. You should always expect at least this minimum of education regarding your disease.

Home-Management Level

Home management goes beyond the above aspects of care. Not only do you learn more about the medication you are receiving, but you also receive more detailed information on products and supplies. In addition, you learn about exercise and about its integral part in your program. It is possible that your health professional will have an exercise prescription developed for you.

Hygiene is also a necessary part of home-management care. This involves hygiene of the hair, the teeth, and the skin, with a specific emphasis on the feet for adults. Your feet get the most punishment of all and therefore need some special care. This includes washing and inspecting your feet daily and then putting on clean socks. Many problems can be avoided if a foot or skin infection is reported to the physician before it has a chance to really become a problem. Unless you have deep skin folds on the sides of your nails, cutting your toenails straight across prevents ingrown toenails and thus a site for infection. Staying away from hot-water bottles, heating pads, and sharp devices also protects those tender feet.

You will learn what to do when you travel, go on vacation,

change your way of life, or become ill. Nausea and vomiting accompany certain types of illnesses; clear liquids containing regular sugar are often recommended during these times, since they are absorbed by the body with greater ease and the energy from the calories helps give you the strength to get well.

You may have difficulty in adjusting to the fact that you have diabetes mellitus. Home management guides you in learning how to handle this adjustment. Perhaps you don't feel like caring for yourself or you are having trouble getting your family's support. You will receive ideas and suggestions on speaking with your family; on finding ways to be appropriately assertive; on finding and using resources to assist you during this period and other times of adjustment.

Learning about the complications of the disease is not done to upset you, but to assist you in making appropriate decisions. If you see that you have an infected toe, getting to the physician so that he or she can assist you in getting your blood-glucose levels as normal as possible, that the toe is treated right away, that you are eating correctly and taking good care of yourself, will most likely mean that the toe will heal faster. The information you receive will assist you in making the more appropriate choices, rather than thinking, "If I'm going to get a complication of diabetes, why try to do anything?"

Self-Management Level

The self-management, or informational, level is the most challenging of all. You will learn not only about how stress affects you, but also about sexuality and diabetes. This level of information helps you to make alterations in your self-care plan. You will learn how to interpret records for patterns or for an individual blood-glucose reading. Learning how to safely self-manage will enable you to have the least number of insulin reactions and yet allow you the tightest control of your diabetes.

This level of information is meant to include in-depth material, more details on what is happening and why. Best yet, it includes what is being done, and why, and what the state of progress is. Knowing is one thing, but taking this information and using it to enhance your diabetes control is another. You will learn when your diabetes management does *not* need to have top priority, and as a result you will have less stress, your blood-glucose levels will become less elevated, and you'll feel better all around.

Choosing an Education Program

How can you identify a quality education program? In the past, this was quite a problem. Today, this is no longer a problem, because a program can be considered high-quality if it has passed the rigors of Self-Recognition (a process developed by the American Diabetes Association, in cooperation with the National Diabetes Advisory Board). This recognition means not only that the staff is recognized as being "acceptable," but also that the program's plan, content, and evaluation process are considered to be within certain specific guidelines. The American Diabetes Association has a list of these programs, which may be obtained either from the national office or from your local chapter.

In such a program, one or more of the staff members are certified diabetes educators (CDEs). A CDE has taken the national board examination and met the qualifications developed by the American Association of Diabetes Educators. The person's experience must have included 2,000 hours of actual practice over at least two years of experience in the field of diabetes education, plus a passing score on a written examination. It does not, of course, mean that this person is perfect! It *does* mean that he or she has a basic knowledge about diabetes, about how to educate another person, and about how to evaluate the process of patient education to see whether success has been achieved.

If your local program and staff members have not yet achieved certification, encourage them to do so. They may already be in the process of applying for recognition. The following topics must be included for a program to be considered for recognition:

Definition of diabetes

Classification

Meal planning

Sick-day care

Medications

Exercise

Hygiene

Travel

Psychological adjustment

New developments

Diabetic ketoacidosis

Neuropathy

Hypoglycemia

Macroangiopathy

Retinopathy

Nephropathy

How Can Education Help You?

Education can help you recognize whether you are receiving up-to-date treatment. It can assist you in making choices on a daily basis. It will help you to know when you should call your health professional, and when it isn't necessary to call. Education will help you feel more confident in your self-care practices. Because you will know where your local and national resources are, if you have a question or need a service you will not need to waste valuable time searching for a resource.

Education can also help your family and friends. They, too, have some adjusting to do. If they do not adjust, you may feel rejected or not supported in the manner that might be most beneficial. If your family and friends learn about diabetes, they will not feel as if they have to "walk on eggshells" when they are around you. They will not have to ask you if you can do this or that or if you can eat this or that. It is true that because they will know what you should do, they may use that information in a nagging way. But if they have truly listened in the classroom and group settings, they will know that nagging is not the thing to do. They will know how best to support you in your endeavor to keep yourself healthy. In fact, they may become healthier as they follow the instructions for the type of health-care program that you are requested to follow. Also, two heads are better than one: when a question arises, you can check with a family member to see whether he or she understood the information given in class in the same way you did.

Most important of all, you should recognize that you are not alone and that there are many, many people interested in your welfare. A good education regarding your diabetes is vital to you and your family. Demand it, and use it.

Chapter 5

Meal Planning

Meal planning involves learning how to choose foods and eating the appropriate amounts. *The so-called diabetic diet is no different from the diet that all people ought to be eating.* It includes plenty of fruits and vegetables; lean meat, chicken, and fish; whole-grain breads and cereals; and low-fat dairy products. The recommended proportions are 30 percent or less fat, 12 to 20 percent protein, and the rest in simple carbohydrates (also called simple sugar) and complex carbohydrates (such as cereals, fruits, and vegetables). (See Appendix A for help in evaluating your own dietary intake.) (Note: the major factor in restricting simple sugars—e.g., table sugar, honey, molasses—is the problem of the body's being unable to get the insulin to the cells in time so that the glucose [or breakdown product of sugar] can enter.)

Basic Eating Guidelines

Much of our life is spent in planning what to eat, preparing food, and eating food. In order for the food to be absorbed, it must be broken into tiny particles. The simpler the food item, the easier it is to absorb. In fact, a few teaspoons of honey given by mouth is absorbed almost as fast as glucose given in the vein. These tiny particles may be completely changed to glucose and have little, if any, nutritional value, or they may contain varying amounts of protein, fat, vitamins, and minerals. Whatever the "food particle," the basic form of storage is glucose.

The three basic food sources are carbohydrates for energy; protein, for cellular growth and repair; fat, for heat and an alternative source of energy. All of these food sources can, to a certain extent, be changed into the carbohydrate glucose, but none of the food sources—including carbohydrates—can be changed into protein. Carbohydrates may be stored as fats (triglycerides), but fats may not be stored as carbohydrates unless they are broken down into parts that include some glucose.

It is recommended that people with diabetes eat a well-balanced diet of nourishing foods that have appropriate nutrients rather than simple sugars having few, if any, important nutrients. Eating the designated portions of these foods at appropriate times will help control the blood-sugar level and maintain the body weight proportionate to the height of the person. Since fat contains a concentrated source of calories, it should be eaten in very limited quantities. To help maintain weight or lose it, if necessary, food intake should be distributed throughout the day into frequent small meals and snacks. This is often patterned into three meals and one or more snacks. The slowest-absorbing food group, protein, should also be distributed appropriately through the day to sustain blood-glucose levels. To aid in digestion and the proper rate of food absorption, a high fiber content is recommended. High-fiber foods include whole-grain breads and cereals, fruits, and vegetables.

The diabetic's diet should thus be made up of nutritious foods containing the needed vitamins and minerals, carbohydrates, proteins, and fats, accompanied by adequate water intake. (See Appendix B for Recommended Dietary Allowances.)

Carbohydrates

Carbohydrates are the body's source of fuel, giving the body energy to be active and to carry on its daily metabolic activities. Carbohydrates contain four calories per gram of weight. Simple carbohydrates are found in simple sugars, such as table sugar, honey, corn syrup, sorghum, date sugar, molasses, brown sugar, powdered sugar, turbinado sugar, and any substance that ends in *-ose* (for example, glucose and fructose).

Complex carbohydrates are cereals, breads, pastas, and vegetables. Fruit contains both simple and complex carbohydrates. Simple carbohydrates are rapidly digested; complex carbohydrates are digested more slowly.

Fats

Fat contains a more concentrated source of calories (with nine calories per gram) than do carbohydrates or protein. Fats carry vitamins and important or essential fatty acids. Examples of fatty foods include butter and margarine, cream, salad dressings, oils, and lard. Some foods, such as avocados, olives, and certain nuts, contain large amounts of fat.

There are five terms in the language of fat that you should know (see Table 5-1). The American Heart Association recommends the use of monounsaturated fats in controlling heart disease.

Cholesterol is a fatlike alcohol found in animal fats and oils. Most of it is developed in the liver, but it can also be absorbed from the diet. Cholesterol is blamed for much of the heart disease

TABLE 5-1

TYPES OF DIETARY FAT

TYPE OF FAT	APPEARANCE AT ROOM TEMP.	EXAMPLE
Saturated	Solid	Butter, lard
Monounsaturated	Liquid	Olive oil
Polyunsaturated	Liquid	Corn oil, safflower oil
Cholesterol	Solid (liquid when heated)	Food derived from animals
Triglycerides*		

*Triglycerides, as their name implies, are made up of three fatty acids bound together by a carbohydrate, sugar alcohol (glycerol).

in our culture. Recent research indicates that it is one of cholesterol's fats—low-density lipoprotein cholesterol (LDL)—that is the bigger culprit. High-density lipoprotein (HDL) cholesterol is the "good guy." Triglyceride in the body is affected by the cholesterol and saturated fat in the diet. When the blood sugar is lowered, the triglyceride level is usually lowered, too.

Proteins

Proteins have four calories per gram and are the most slowly absorbed foods. Until the early 1980s, fats were considered to be the slowest-absorbing of the three food groups. Research from a university on the East coast determined otherwise. Proteins have a greater than 50 percent capability of being changed into glucose. While fats must be changed into ketone bodies before being used as an energy source, proteins need only to be changed into glucose.

All animal sources contain protein. This includes dairy products, meats, and fish. Vegetable plant sources contain protein, but in varying amounts. Grains also contain protein.

Other Nutrients

Other nutrients are also important in meeting the needs of the human body. Nutrients are found both in minerals (such as iron and calcium) and in vitamins (as in A, B_1, B_2, B_3, C, D, and so forth). Along with the three food groups, nutrients are needed as an energy source and are used for growth and repair of body tissue. Although there are roughly fifty nutrients needed for daily growth and development, only the major vitamins and minerals are discussed here.

Iron is the carrier of oxygen to body tissues. Anemia is prevented through adequate iron in the diet. Calcium is used for building strong bones and teeth; it is also used in muscle contraction and relaxation and in the proper functioning of the nerves. Vitamin A is known for its role in promoting good vision. Its lesser but still important role is in keeping the skin and mucous membranes in good condition.

Vitamin B_1 aids in digestion and in muscle and nerve function. B_2 helps in promoting healthy skin and mucous membranes and general vitality. B$_3$ aids in digestion, keeping the nerves and skin in good condition. Vitamin C has many more roles than was thought earlier. It helps not only in the healing processes but also in maintaining healthy gums, bones, tissues, blood, and blood vessels. Vitamin D assists in the utilization of calcium and in the maintenance of healthy bones.

Baseline Meal Planning

Meal plans are made to help you rather than to be an obstacle. They should be individualized to meet your particular needs, wants, and lifestyle and organized within the bounds of your particular health problem(s). The plan must meet the calorie level of your daily activity, unless you are overweight, in which case you need to decrease your caloric intake in relation to the calories you burn in daily activity (with a weight-loss goal of from one-half to two pounds per week).

The three most important things to keep in mind are these:

1. Be sure that you are getting the nutrition you need to meet your energy demands.

2. The food should be distributed throughout the day so that the body is not overwhelmed at any one time.

3. The food pattern and amounts eaten should be consistent, unless a greater or lesser energy use requires a greater or lesser amount of food intake.

The purpose of a meal plan is to help you achieve these important goals.

A meal plan may be developed using a variety of methods. To figure out the ideal body weight for a female, take the height (for example, 5'4") and give 100 pounds for the first five feet and 5 pounds for each inch above five feet. That would be 100 + (4 × 5), for an ideal body weight of 120 pounds for a medium-boned female, plus or minus 10 percent to allow for differences in bone structure (that is, large-boned or small-boned). For males, 106 pounds are given for the first five feet of height, and 6 pounds for each inch above five feet. For a male who is 5'11" tall, the calculations would be 106 + (11 × 6) = 172 pounds, plus or minus 10 percent to account for bone structure.

The average recommended dietary intake is 10–15 calories per pound (20–30 calories per kilogram), depending on whether you are male or female and active or inactive. A pregnant woman requires up to 17 calories per pound (39 calories/kg), especially during the last trimester; nursing mothers also require this amount. An infant needs roughly 55 calories per pound, and a school-age child needs 30 or more.

These calories need to be distributed throughout the day in a pattern of three meals and one to three between-meal snacks. Children, especially, thrive on three meals and three snacks. Because their stomachs are too small to hold larger quantities at mealtimes and their ability to store glucose is limited because of their size, some food intake every two or three hours is most appropriate. As they grow, children need an increase in caloric intake to meet their needs. This can be figured scientifically with a chart or mathematic calculation. It can also be done by noting when the child is consistently eating more than the baseline meal plan that was calculated in the office or hospital, and then increasing the total meal plan by that extra number of calories (usually in increments of 100 or 200 calories).

The goal of any meal plan is to meet caloric and nutritional requirements with high-fiber, low-fat foods, with little or no concentrated sweets. The meal plan should be altered for changes in growth, activity level, and lifestyle.

The three major approaches to meal planning are constant carbohydrate, the exchange lists (composed of six food groups—see Appendix C), and food points (see Appendixes D and E). Constant carbohydrate means that a person is requested to eat so many servings of carbohydrate foods to equal a certain number of grams of carbohydrate. Little restriction is placed on fat and protein other than following the recommended dietary intake of 12–15 percent protein, 30 percent or less fat, and the rest in carbohydrates. The exchange lists are noted in detail in the appendixes.

The food-points system was first planned for a non–English-speaking population. It can be used to plan for a certain amount of carbohydrates, protein, fat, major vitamins and minerals, cholesterol, sodium, and calories. We use the calorie system (75 calories = 1 point). The food is distributed throughout the day in serving sizes. Some of the more common distributions are noted in Table 5-2.

TABLE 5-2

STANDARD CALORIE-POINT DISTRIBUTION

3 MEALS AND 3 SNACKS

CALORIES	CALORIE POINTS	BREAKFAST 4/18	MORNING SNACK 1/18	LUNCH 5/18	AFTERNOON SNACK 2/18	EVENING MEAL 5/18	BEDTIME SNACK 1/18
			(OF TOTAL CALORIE INTAKE)				
1000	13.5	3	1	3.5	1.5	3.5	1
1200	16	3.5	1	4.5	1.5	4.5	1
1400	18.5	4	1	5	2	5.5	1
1600	21.5	5	1	6	2	6	1.5
1800	24	5.5	1.5	6.5	2.5	6.5	1.5
2000	26.5	6	1.5	7	3	7	2
2500	33.5	7.5	2	9	3.5	9.5	2
3000	40	9	2	11	4.5	11.5	2

Special Needs

If weight loss is needed, the meal plan will need to be changed. It takes the equivalent of just one extra slice of bread per day to result in a pound of weight gain in a month. Weight loss requires following these rules:

1. The intake must be less than the energy output.

2. The food intake must be distributed throughout the day.

3. Food intake should be limited to the daylight hours, and food should not be eaten later than two to three hours before bedtime unless the person is on insulin (in which case there should be a bedtime snack).

4. A vitamin supplement is recommended if the total caloric level is below 1200 calories/day. (Any plan below this level will have difficulty meeting the recommended daily requirements of vitamins and minerals.)

5. Liquid-protein diets are recommended only for the greatly overweight person, and any person using such products should be closely monitored by a physician.

6. An exercise program must be carried out on a daily or every-other-day basis.

Elevation in cholesterol or triglycerides requires a careful monitoring and restriction of fat intake (and, especially for triglycerides, restriction of alcohol intake). Again, exercise is helpful for both of these conditions. For triglyceride problems, the normalization of blood-glucose levels is helpful. If hyperlipidemia (high fat content in the blood) is a genetic rather than a dietary problem, the physician will prescribe appropriate medication dosages to assist in normalizing the cholesterol and/or triglyceride levels.

Hypertension (high blood pressure) may require a decrease in salt intake. This problem may be due to diabetic kidney disease or to other factors, such as age and weight. If you have complications from your diabetes, hypertension may aggravate these. In any case, normalizing your blood pressure is accomplished by taking the medication prescribed by your physician and eating nutritiously, both in amounts and choices. Keep the salt shaker off the table. Refrain from eating salty foods such as hot dogs, TV dinners, most canned soups, and potato chips. Although salt substitutes may be used, fresh foods usually contain enough sodium chloride (table salt) for body needs.

Preventing hypoglycemia means that you need to carry some form of simple sugar or food with you at all times. Foods to carry might be dried fruits or preprocessed packets of crackers. Granola bars or small cans of juice would also be helpful to have at hand. These foods could be used when there is an unexpected increase in activity level, for planned extra activity, or when low blood-glucose levels need treatment (that is, when blood sugar is higher than 40 mg/dl [2 mMol]). Below that level, simple sugar is needed.

Food intake during illness varies. If someone is experiencing nausea, with or without vomiting, clear liquids will be needed. Some health professionals recommend that the clear liquids not contain any sugar until the blood-glucose levels are below 300 mg/dl (17 mMol). Others say that the calories are still needed for the energy requirement to combat the illness, with insulin supplements given to compensate for the elevation in blood-glucose levels. Almost all physicians agree that during an illness accompanied by nausea, vomiting, and diarrhea, a patient with blood-glucose levels in the 200 mg/dl (11 mMol) range or less requires clear, sugar-containing liquids for twenty-four to forty-eight hours. The person may then progress to eating crackers and dry toast. If the crackers and toast are tolerated, soups and other light foods may be tried.

If the activity level is decreased, then fewer total calories are needed. For illness, the usual recommendation is to take 20 percent fewer total calories than you usually need on an active day. This level would be increased when the activity returns to its usual level. The principles to remember are these:

1. Fewer calories are needed when the body is at rest.

2. Simpler foods are easier to digest.

3. Fluid intake (noncaloric or low-calorie beverages) should be encouraged unless nausea, vomiting, and diarrhea are present.

4. *If in doubt, contact your health professional.*

Each different change in health level or activity level needs individual attention at the time of the change. If you have *not* been educated to make the appropriate changes, contact your health professional for advice.

Chapter 6

Diabetes Medication

Many people who have diabetes mellitus need one of two types of medication to control their blood-glucose levels. One type of medication assists in the use and availability of insulin, while the other medication actually replaces the body's lost insulin-making ability. The choice depends on the body's response. For people with Type II diabetes, if the average blood-glucose levels are greater than 150 mg/dl (8 mMol), then an oral hypoglycemic agent is needed. Unless what is going on in your body suggests otherwise (e.g., you are unable or unwilling to lose weight, or your blood sugar is high in spite of weight loss), you need this type of diabetes medication (see Table 6-1).

If the oral agent used at the maximum dosage is not effective (that is, if it is unable to lower blood sugars below 180 mg/dl [10 mMol]), then insulin is needed. In some cases, insulin and a second-generation oral hypoglycemic agent are combined.

Oral Hypoglycemic Agents

Oral hypoglycemic agents are not insulin "pills" but powdered, compressed medications that appear to affect the

TABLE 6-1

ORAL HYPOGLYCEMIC AGENTS

First-Generation Drugs:	Tolbutamide	(Orinase)
	Acetohexamide	(Dymelor)
	Tolazamide	(Tolinase)
	Chlorpropamide	(Diabinese)
Second-Generation Drugs:	Glyburide	(Micronase, DiaBeta, Glynase)
	Glipizide	(Glucotrol, Glucotrol XL)

---

insulin-making ability of the beta cells of the pancreas, stimulate the forming of receptor sites on the cells, correct some post receptor defects on the insides of the cells, and effect production of glucose by the liver (hepatic glucose production).

You must have some insulin-making ability to be able to respond to an oral agent. If your body is not making enough insulin or the cells in your body are not able to correctly use the insulin you are making, and if simple control of dietary intake (or getting your body weight closer to normal) is not effective, you probably need an oral agent to help control your blood-glucose levels. If this does not work for you, then another choice of medication is made.

Many people think that if they are taking the pills they do not need to watch their dietary intake. This is not true. You must still eat spaced meals and one or more snacks each day and follow all the other parts of your self-care program. It is also important to check your blood-glucose levels to be sure that the medication is working to meet the goal of premeal blood-glucose levels of between 70–110 mg/dl (4–6 mMol) and two-hour postmeal (postprandial) levels of less than 150 mg/dl (8 mMol) (or at least less than 180 mg/dl [10 mMol]).

You must also be knowledgeable about the side effects of oral agents. These are hypoglycemia (low blood sugar), nausea, and vomiting. Yellowing of the skin (jaundice) and skin rashes have also been reported. Except for hypoglycemia, these side effects occur in fewer than 1 percent of people taking these medications.

You need to be familiar with the interaction of your diabetes medication with any other medications you might be taking. Drinking alcohol while you are taking chlorpropamide may result in an Antabuse type of reaction (flushing of the skin, nausea, and vomiting). With the first-generation oral hypoglycemic agents, taking another drug during the same day may cause either the drug or the oral agents to work more or less effectively. Drugs that may interact with these agents include anticoagulants, birth-control pills, diuretics, steroids, and Dilantin (which raise the blood sugar), as well as some that lower blood sugar, including aspirin and some medicines used to treat high blood pressure (such as Inderal). Oral agents are not prescribed for children or for women who are pregnant or breast-feeding. If you are ill or having surgery, the physician may choose to have you take insulin for a period of time. You also need to be familiar with the time action of the oral hypoglycemic agents. This allows you to either predict or determine the potential for hypoglycemic episodes.

Short-Acting Agents

There is only one short-acting oral agent. It is called tolbutamide (the generic name) or Orinase (the brand name). If the physician places the generic name on the prescription, you can often receive the product at its lowest cost. The generic pill is available in 500-mg tablets from the Barr, Danbury, Lederle, and Zenith drug companies. It starts working in one hour and is half-used in about 5.6 hours; the total time it works in the body is approximately 6 to 12 hours. The recommended dosage is no more than three grams (or six 500-mg tablets) per day.

Intermediate-Acting Agents

The intermediate-acting oral agents are acetohexamide (Dymelor) and tolazamide (Tolinase) from the first generation, and glipizide (Glucotrol) and glyburide (Micronase or DiaBeta) from the second generation (see Table 6-1). The first-generation pills were tested and put on the market in the 1950s and 1960s. The second-generation pills were tested in the United States and put on the market in the 1970s and 1980s.

ACETOHEXAMIDE (DYMELOR) Acetohexamide (Dymelor) comes in 250-mg and 500-mg tablets and is available from the Eli Lilly Pharmaceutical Company. This medication starts working in about one hour, and over half of its usefulness occurs within five hours. It lasts in the body for approximately ten to fourteen hours. The maximum dosage recommended is 1.5 grams (six of the 250-mg tablets or three of the 500-mg tablets) per day. If you have problems with improper functioning of your kidneys, this would not be a medication that your doctor would recommend.

TOLAZAMIDE (TOLINASE) Tolazamide (Tolinase) is an oral agent that is absorbed more slowly (its onset is four to six hours). If you have a tendency to absorb food slowly, then this oral agent might be recommended for you. It comes in 100-mg, 250-mg, and 500-mg tablets, from the Upjohn Company. Half of the usefulness of this medication in your body occurs within approximately seven hours. The maximum recommended dosage is one gram (ten 100-mg tablets, four 250-mg tablets, or two 500-mg tablets) per day. This product is also available as a generic through the Barr, Danbury, Lederle, and Zenith companies.

GLYBURIDE Glyburide is a product available through the Upjohn Company (Micronase and Glynase) and the Hoechst-Roussel Company (DiaBeta). The tablet sizes are 1.25 mg, 2.5 mg, and 5 mg. The maximum dose recommended is 20 mg/day. Glynase is a more bioactive drug (i.e. works slightly better). It is available in 3 mg and 6 mg tablets. These tablets are easily broken into two pieces. As with any other intermediate-acting oral agent, the dosages are usually divided (some before breakfast and some before supper) when 10 mg or more of medication are needed. The onset is 1.5 hours, and the total duration is around 24 hours. Half of the medication's usefulness may occur anywhere from 3.2 hours, for part of its chemical action, to up to 10 hours for the rest of its half-life. Half of this medication is excreted in the urine and the other half through the bile in the liver, but caution is still encouraged for use in the elderly.

GLIPIZIDE (GLUCOTROL) Glipizide (Glucotrol) is a 5-mg or 10-mg tablet product developed by Pfizer but marketed by Roerig Company. It is documented as being more slowly absorbed, but its action begins an hour after it is swallowed. The half-life is 3.5 to 6 hours, and it may remain in the body for anywhere from 12 to 16 hours. It is recommended that a total of no more than 40 mg be taken in a day, and that the medication should be taken on an empty stomach (that is, about thirty minutes before a meal). If more than 15 mg are needed, the dose should be divided. Glucotrol XL has more recently been made available. The XL stands for extended life or longer lasting medication. The top dose of Glucotrol XL is 20 mg. Although this medication is changed in the liver to an inactive form, caution for use in the elderly is recommended.

Long-Acting Agents

There is only one long-acting oral agent. This medication is also of the first generation and should not be used by anyone who has problems with kidney function or fluid retention. It should also be used with caution in the elderly. Chlorpropamide (Diabinese) is a product of the Pfizer Company. It is available in 100-mg and 250-mg tablets. The maximum dose recommended is 500 mg (five 100-mg tablets or two 250-mg tablets) per day. It has the longest half-life, with thirty-five hours, but its action starts in about an hour. The duration of this medication in the body is around seventy-two hours. An antidiuretic type of effect may lead to fluid retention and low salt (sodium) levels in the body.

General Recommendations

Oral hypoglycemic agents have their place in the medical management of diabetes, but when the blood sugar is no longer controlled by the maximum recommended amount of medication, there is no other recourse than to administer life-saving insulin. If more of the oral agent is taken than is recommended, it is very possible that the person could become quite sick.

Insulin

Before insulin was discovered, a child who had diabetes could expect to live only about two years, on average, from the time of diagnosis. Insulin was first chemically removed from the pancreases of animals, but human insulin may now be made semisynthetically from pork insulin or biologically engineered using recombinant-DNA technology. These forms of insulin (animal, semisynthetic, or biosynthetic) are available on the pharmacy shelves. As more of the semisynthetic and biologically engineered insulin becomes available, less and less of the animal-derived insulin (highly purified pork or beef or a pork/beef mix) will be used.

Like oral hypoglycemic agents, insulin is available in short-acting, intermediate-acting, and long-acting forms (see Table 6-2).

Lente (L) is a premixed, crystalline, intermediate-acting insulin. The short-acting form of this type of insulin is called Semilente (S), and it contains numerous small crystals. The long-acting form, Ultralente (U), contains a smaller number of crystals, but they are larger in size. Lente insulin is a mixture of the two types (30 percent Semilente and 70 percent Ultralente), but because of the slower onset of action of the Semilente insulin, it is often mixed with short-action (or rapid-action, or Regular) insulin to get a quicker early action along with later action.

TABLE 6-2

LIST OF INSULINS

ELI LILLY INSULINS

TYPE OF INSULIN	SOURCE
SHORT-ACTING (Therapeutic action: onset 15–30 minutes, peak 2–4 hours, duration 6–8 hours)	
Iletin II R	Pork (purified)
Iletin I R	Pork & Beef
Humulin R	Human
Humulin BR	Human (for pumps)
INTERMEDIATE-ACTING (Therapeutic action: onset 2 hours, peak 4–12 hours, duration 10–14 hours)	
Iletin I N	Pork & Beef
Iletin II N	Pork (purified)
Humulin N	Human
(Therapeutic action: onset 2 hours, peak 8–12 hours, duration 12–16 hours)	
Iletin I L	Pork & Beef
Iletin II L	Pork (purified)
Humulin L	Human
LONG-ACTING (Therapeutic action: onset 8 hours, peak 18 hours, duration 24–36 hours)	
Iletin I U	Human

TYPE OF INSULIN	SOURCE

(Therapeutic action: onset 15–30 minutes/2 hours, peak 2–12 hours, duration 6–12 hours) (Humulin 70/30 is a mixture of 30% Regular and 70% NPH, 50/50 is a mixture of 50% Regular and 50% NPH)

Humulin 70/30	Human
Humulin 50/50	Human

NOVO-NORDISK INSULINS

TYPE OF INSULIN	SOURCE

SHORT-ACTING (Therapeutic action: onset 15–30 minutes, peak 2–4 hours, duration 6–8 hours)

Regular	Pork (Purified)
Novolin R	Human

INTERMEDIATE-ACTING (Therapeutic action: onset 2 hours, peak 4–12 hours, duration 10–14 hours)

NPH	Beef & Pork (purified)
Novolin N	Human

(Therapeutic action: onset 2 hours, peak 8–12 hours, duration 12–16 hours)

Lente	Beef
Novolin L	Human

TYPE OF INSULIN	SOURCE

LONG-ACTING (Therapeutic action: onset 8 hours, peak 18 hours, duration 24–36 hours)

Ultralente	Beef

(Therapeutic action: onset 15–30 minutes/2 hours, peak 2–12 hours, duration 6–12 hours) (All are mixtures of 30% Regular and 70% NPH)

Novolin 70/30	Human

When a protein called protamine is attached to a short acting insulin, it becomes NPH (Neutral Protamine Hagedorn [N]), an intermediate-acting insulin. The insulin of the future (called designer or "tailored" insulin) will have some of the proteins in the insulin chain changed in their sequence. This will result in the effect of the time action of insulin.

The major side effects that can occur when taking insulin are as follows:

low blood sugar

hypoglycemia (also called insulin reaction or insulin shock)

lipodystrophy (a change in the fatty tissue under the skin)

hypertrophy (an enlarged area that results from receiving the shot in the same place for too long)

atrophy (a sunken area, as a response to the insulin and its diluting agent; has been observed less frequently with the advent of human insulin)

Other side effects may be a rash at the site of the injection or a rash all over the body. However, these and other side effects are seldom noted.

In the United States, insulin is available in a concentration of 100 units per 1 cc, called U100 (or the seldom-used U40). For special purposes, such as research, U400 and U500 are available. Most other countries are currently in the process of converting their available insulin into the U100 form. (Note: some U40 or U80 insulin may be more readily available in other parts of the world.)

If a child or adult is extremely sensitive to insulin changes, then the insulin may be diluted to be U50 (a 1:1 dilution) or U25 (a 1:3 dilution—one part insulin with three parts diluting fluid). This allows changes in the insulin dosage in ¼- to ½-unit changes rather than 1-unit changes. The syringes, such as the 50-unit, syringe (or the 30-unit syringe) allow the careful measuring of single unit changes. Therefore, diluting insulin may not be needed.

As with your meal plan, the insulin is spaced throughout the day to enable your body to handle your food intake in relation to your activity pattern. Therefore, the time action of the insulin is very important. When you look at a chart or read about the time action of insulin, notice whether it is concerned with the phar-macokinetic or therapeutic (effective) action of insulin. The phar-macokinetic action (also called the pharmacologic action) of in-sulin is the response of the body to the insulin from the time it enters the body until it is no longer measurable in the body. The therapeutic (effective) duration of action of the insulin is the time a certain amount of insulin will keep your blood-sugar level within the normal range (see Table 6-3). The former is important to scientists but the latter is more important to the patients.

To keep your blood-sugar and insulin levels within the nor-mal range, you must know how the insulin performs therapeutic-ally (refer back to Table 6-2).

Two companies, Eli Lilly and Novo-Nordisk Pharmaceuti-cals, are currently producing insulin in the United States. They, as well as other professionals in the field, are recognizing that there is seldom a case when one dose of insulin will cover the twenty-four-hour needs of the person who has diabetes. Es-pecially with human insulins, the three-dose program is being used more frequently. Twenty-four-hour control of the blood-glucose level is the goal. If less is achieved, problems are more apt to occur. The body normally produces a small amount of insulin continuously—basal insulin—and a burst of insulin with each intake of food. It is this pattern that needs to be duplicated with injectable insulin if control over the whole twenty-four-hour period is to be achieved.

TABLE 6-3

THERAPEUTIC GOALS FOR BLOOD SUGARS

Premeal: 60–120 mg/dl (3–7 mMol)

2 hrs. after a meal: less than 150 mg/dl (8 mMol)

For the pregnant woman (and, ideally, for others as they can tolerate it):

Premeal: 70–100 mg/dl (4–6 mMol)

2 hrs. after a meal: less than 120 mg/dl (7 mMol), or at least less than
                    130 mg/dl (7 mMol)

(Average blood sugars should be 90–100 md/dl [5–6 mMol])

Short-Acting Insulin

The short-acting insulins are Regular, Velosulin, Iletin II R, Iletin I R, Novolin R, or Humulin R. These insulins start working within thirty minutes, with the strongest—or peak—action occurring in two to four hours. The pharmacokinetic duration of action is from six to eight hours or longer, while the therapeutic duration of action is between four and eight hours. (Note: Semilente insulins are no longer available in the United States as of February, 1994.)

Intermediate-Acting Insulin

The intermediate-acting insulins are NPH, Purified Pork N, Iletin II NPH, Iletin I NPH, Novolin N, Humulin NPH, Iletin II Lente, Iletin I Lente, Novolin L (human), and Humulin L. These start working in one to two hours, with peak action in four to twelve hours. The pharmacokinetic duration of action is reported to be twenty-four hours (the shortest therapeutic action reported is ten to sixteen hours). (Note that the human NPH insulins have a therapeutic duration of action closer to ten hours, while the pork or beef/pork Lente insulins have an action closer to sixteen hours.)

Long-Acting Insulin

Long-acting insulin has been playing a newer role in the management of diabetes. This insulin—Iletin (Ultralente) has what is termed a "flat curve." Instead of rising to a certain point and then dropping off, the action results in an elevated rise that remains for a long time before the effect is decreased. Since this duration is greater than twenty-four hours, an overlapping effect creates a continued blood level. The long-acting insulin is Iletin IU (human). This insulin takes much longer to act (about eight hours), peaks in about eighteen hours, and has a pharmacokinetic action of thirty-six hours or more. Its therapeutic actions are about twenty-four to thirty-six hours (even, in the past, reported as up to seventy-two hours for nonhuman insulin). They are often used in the so-called "poor man's pump-management program." This is really a misnomer, but it is a useful term. The long-acting insulins are used for a basal insulin effect (a little insulin every so many minutes), with doses (called "boluses") of short-acting insulin given prior to each meal or large snack. This is a very effective way for some individuals to manage their diabetes.

Premixed Insulin

Premixed insulins are now being used more frequently. Eli Lilly has a 70/30 human mixture (70 percent NPH and 30 percent R-Humulin 70/30), as does Novo-Nordisk (Mixtard—pork or human, and Novolin 70/30—human; penfill cartridges and prefilled cartridges). 50/50 insulin has been developed and is available for use (Europe has other combinations of insulin in addition to 70/30 and 50/50). So far, the Food and Drug Administration has only approved the 70/30 and the 50/50 mixture.

Methods of Insulin Delivery

Insulin may be delivered in one of a number of ways: under the skin (subcutaneously), into the muscle (intramuscularly), or into the vein (intravenously). The instrument used for delivery of insulin may be a syringe/needle, syringe autoinjector, hydrospray injector, IV infusion equipment, or insulin infusion pump. Subcutaneous insulin is given only by syringe, autoinjector, or hyprospray. When insulin is administered in any other way (by vein, into the muscle, or with an infusion pump), only the short-acting insulin is given. The fastest way to receive insulin is through an injection into the vein. The next-fastest way is to have it delivered by syringe and needle into the muscle. The peak action of intramuscular insulin is about one and a half hours, rather than the two to four hours for insulin injected under the skin.

The important points about giving insulin subcutaneously are to ensure the cleanliness of the process and to give the correct amount at the right time (see Table 6-4). All parts of the procedure are important. However, while omitting certain steps will not have a detrimental effect on the blood-glucose levels, omitting some other steps will. When getting insulin out of the bottle, first clean the top of the bottle, then replace the vacuum in which the insulin is placed by injecting into the bottle an amount of air that is equal to the amount of insulin to be removed. To be sure the

TABLE 6-4

STEPS IN INSULIN INJECTION

1. Wash hands.
2. Clean bottle top.
3. Pull air into bottle from syringe.
4. Push air into bottle from syringe.
5. Pull insulin into syringe (bubble free).
6. Clean skin.
7. Inject needle (45–90° angle).
8. Pull needle out.
9. Mild pressure on site.

---

correct amount of insulin is injected, you can do the following: check that the amount of air to be injected into the bottle is equal to the amount of insulin to be removed, check the amount of insulin in the syringe in relation to the dosage to be given, and check the syringe against the bottle to make sure that you have placed the insulin from that specific bottle into the syringe.

To assure that the right bottle is chosen at the right time, color-code the labels (for example, red for morning mixture, green for the Regular at suppertime, and blue for the bedtime NPH dose).

Mixing Insulins for Injection

If insulin is to be mixed in a syringe (see Table 6-5), the tops of both bottles are cleansed, and air equal to the insulin to be removed is injected into each of the bottles. Once the air is placed into the short-acting insulin bottle (e.g., Regular), the desired amount of insulin is withdrawn. The needle is removed from that bottle and carefully placed into the other bottle. The insulin is very carefully withdrawn until the total amount of dosage is obtained in the syringe (for example, ten units of Regular plus

TABLE 6-5

STEPS IN MIXING INSULIN IN A SYRINGE

1. Wash hands.
2. Wipe off tops of both bottles.
3. Pull air into syringe, equal to insulin desired.
4. Push air into bottles from syringe.
5. Pull insulin into syringe (bubble free) from bottle #1 (for example, Regular).
6. Pull insulin into syringe (bubble free) to total mark from bottle #2 (for example, NPH).
7. Clean skin.
8. Inject needle (45–90° angle).
9. Pull needle out.
10. Mild pressure on site.

---

twenty units of NPH drawn up, in total, to the thirty-unit mark on the syringe).

This insulin should be administered within five minutes from the time it was initially mixed. If the insulin is premixed in separate syringes or in a mixing bottle, it is necessary to wait fifteen minutes before administering that insulin dosage from the syringe or bottle. Premixed insulin should not be kept in a syringe for longer than two weeks.

Premixing of Lente with Regular insulin is not recommended unless it is administered immediately. Lente insulins cannot be premixed with NPH or PZI insulins. Premixed NPH and Regular are now available as 70/30 mixes and are usable up to the date (shelf life) on the box.

The least amount of discomfort is experienced during the injection when the insulin is at room or body temperature and is given without any "drag" on the needle (that is, the needle must either pierce tight skin or be rapidly placed through the skin layer). Insulin in use can be kept at room temperature for up to three months. However, if kept at a temperature greater than 90° or below 32°F, the insulin may be damaged.

To prevent infection, the skin should be as clean as possible. To be sure of this, give the injection after a bath or shower, or wash the injection area with soap and water or with a cleansing wipe. The skin should be made tight by pinching a large fold of skin or, in the case of loose skin (such as might be found on the abdomen), pinching and stretching the skin so that the injection will be given in the stretched area, not the pinched area.

The injection is given at an angle of forty-five to ninety degrees, unless atrophy is to be treated, in which case a twenty-degree angle is recommended. The angle depends on the thickness of the skin. In other words, a younger child or elderly person would most likely need a forty-five-degree angle injection, while a young or middle-aged adult would probably need a ninety-degree angle. Once the insulin has been administered at an even rate of speed, the needle should be quickly withdrawn at the same angle at which it was inserted. Mild pressure on the injection site for a period of a minute or less will aid in keeping the insulin from leaking out onto the skin surface. (Some people use what is called Z-tracking: The needle is placed through the skin, the tip is moved to an angle, and the insulin is pushed in. On removal, the tip is moved back to its original location and is then pulled from the body. Such a technique is not usually necessary, but can be helpful for those who experience a lot of "leaking.")

Other Methods of Insulin Delivery

A number of other methods of insulin delivery are available (see Table 6-6).

Autoinjectors (Busher Automatic Injector, Injectomatic, Autojector, Inject-ease, Instaject I, Instaject II, Monoject) may assist in getting the needle through the skin, with the person either pushing the plunger in to administer the insulin or shooting both the needle and the insulin into the skin. The cost varies from $20 to $150. The jet injectors (Medi-Jector II, Medi-Jector EZ, Medi-Jector, Tender Touch, Preci-Jet 50, and Vitajet II) will blow the insulin through the skin. The depth may be regulated through adjustments of the nozzle of the jet injector unit. Proper cleaning

TABLE 6-6

INJECTION DEVICES

PRODUCT/ MANUFACTURER	APPROXIMATE PRICE	WARRANTY	COMMENTS
AUTOMATIC INJECTORS			
INJECT-EASE Palco Laboratories 1595 Soquel Drive Santa Cruz, CA 95065 (800) 346-4488	$25–$30	Five years, plus money-back guarantee	Uses B-D, Terumo, Pharmaplast, and EZ-Ject syringes
INJECTOMATIC Sherwood Medical; distributed by Kendall Futuro 5801 Mariemont Ave. Cincinnati, OH 45227 (800) 543-4452	$20–$30	One year, plus 30-day, money-back guarantee	Uses Monoject syringes only
INSTAJECT Jordan Enterprises 12555 Garden Grove Blvd. Suite 507 Garden Grove, CA 92643 (800) 541-1193	$50	One year, plus 30-day money-back guarantee	Uses all brands and sizes of disposable syringes

PRODUCT/ MANUFACTURER	APPROXIMATE PRICE	WARRANTY	COMMENTS
AUTOMATIC NEEDLE AND INSULIN INJECTORS			
AUTOJECTOR Ulster Scientific, Inc. P.O. Box 902 Highland, NY 12528 NY State: (800) 522-2257 Outside NY: (800) 341-8233	$40	Two years, plus 30-day, money-back guarantee	Uses most brands and sizes of disposable syringes
DIAMATIC Ulster Scientific, Inc. P.O. Box 902 Highland, NY 12528 NY State: (800) 522-2257 Outside NY: (800) 341-8233	$130	Two years	Uses most brands and sizes of disposable syringes
PEN INJECTORS			
NOVOLINPEN (disposable) NovoNordisk Pharmaceuti- cals, Inc. 100 Overlook Center, Suite 200 Princeton, NJ 08540 (800) 223-0872	$40	One year	Uses 27-gauge needle. Delivers 2 units to 36 units in even dosages only.

PRODUCT/ MANUFACTURER	APPROXIMATE PRICE	WARRANTY	COMMENTS
NOVOPEN NovoNordisk Pharmaceuticals, Inc. 100 Overlook Center, Suite 200 Princeton, NJ 08540 (800) 223-0872	$95	One year	Uses 27-gauge needle. Delivers even and odd dosages.
AUTOPEN Owen Mumford; distributed by Ulster Scientific, Inc. P.O. Box 902 Highland, NY 12528 NY State: (800) 522-2257 Outside NY: (800) 341-8233	$45	One year	Uses 27-gauge needle. Delivers up to 32 units in even dosages only.
JET INJECTORS MEDI-JECTOR EZ Derata Corp. 1840 Berkshire Lane Minneapolis, MN 55441 (800) 328-3074	$595	Three years, plus 30-day prorated money-back guarantee	Delivers 2 units to 50 units; prescription required.

PRODUCT/ MANUFACTURER	APPROXIMATE PRICE	WARRANTY	COMMENTS
MEDI-JECTOR II Derata Corp. 1840 Berkshire Lane Minneapolis, MN 55441 (800) 328-3074	$795	Five years, plus 30-day prorated money-back guarantee	Delivers 2 units to 100 units; prescription required.
TENDER TOUCH Derata Corp. 1840 Berkshire Lane Minneapolis, MN 55441 (800) 328-3074	$595	Three years, plus 30-day, prorated money-back guarantee	Delivers 1 unit to 50 units; prescription required.
VITAJET PRECISION INSTRUMENTS, INC. Mada Equipment Co. 600 Commerce Rd. Carlstadt, NJ 07072 (800) 848-2538	$689	Two years	Delivers ½ unit to 50 units; prescription required.

Adapted from Peragallo-Dittko V. 1990. "Buyer's Guide to Injection Devices." *Diabetes Self Management,* Jan.–Feb., 6–7, 9–12.

of the mechanism through which the insulin is blown is a necessary step in the use of these instruments. Costs range from about $500 to $900. Bottles or vials of insulin are used (see Figure 6-1).

With the insulin pens (Accupen, NovoPen, and Novolinpen), vials or cartridges are usually used. Figure 6-2 shows the changes that have occurred in insulin pen injectors. These pens are available through Ulster Scientific and Novo-Nordisk Pharmaceutical, Inc. The cost is from $40 to $100.

FIGURE 6-1

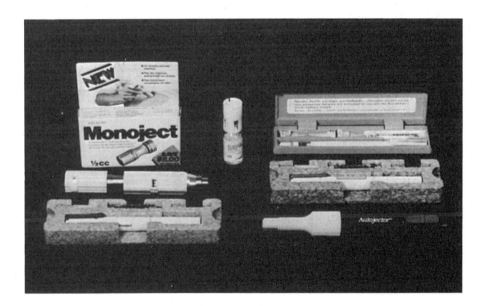

FIGURE 6-2

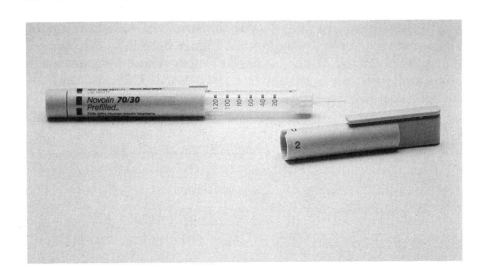

The Button Infuser (Markwell Medical Institute) and Insulflon (Diabetes Center, Inc.) aid in multiple-injection therapy. The multiple daily injections are given through a diaphragm connected to tubing that has been placed beneath the skin. This placement is usually done on a weekly basis.

CPI, Minimed, and Medix Medical Electronics are the companies that have or are making insulin infusion pumps (see Figure 6-3). These highly technical instruments administer a basal insulin (insulin at certain small intervals throughout a twenty-four-hour period), plus an automatic or manual dose before each meal or at other desired times. Individuals using these instruments must be knowledgeable, stable, and motivated. For safety's sake, blood-glucose tests must be taken four to six times or more a day. This is truly a case in which more is not better: having consistently lower-than-normal blood-glucose levels means that fewer physical signals will be felt if the blood-sugar level drops even further. It also means that the body has not had the opportunity to attain and maintain stored glucose for emergency use, so little backup sugar will be available if the blood-sugar level

FIGURE 6-3

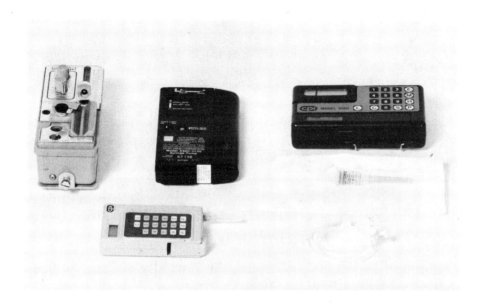

goes even lower. The Minimed 506 and Disetronic's H-Tron V-100 are, at present, the only infusion pumps sold in the United States. Plugging of the tubing, lack of battery power, and running out of insulin from the vial or syringe are some of the potential problems. Humulin BR and velo-sulin human (buffered) have helped decrease the first problem; regarding the second, the machine usually has a signal to let the wearer know that the battery needs changing. Pumps will become safer and more usable as these machines are refined, and especially if a glucose sensor is developed that can signal the machine as to how much insulin is needed. It is quite possible that in the future, these pumps will be used by a greater number of people (see Figure 6-4 for an example of a pump). At present, the same level of management can be achieved with the use of multiple doses of insulin, at a much lower cost.

FIGURE 6-4

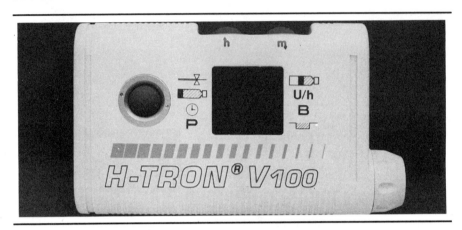

Special Instruments for Insulin Administration

Equipment is available to assist the partially sighted or blind individual in reading the syringe (Insul-eze, Magni-Guide, and Syringe Magnified). These may be purchased either through the American Foundation for the Blind or directly from the manufacturer. Instruments that aid in getting the appropriate dosage into the syringe are Adros IDM, Click-Count, Count-a-Dose, Dose-Aid, Insulgage, Holdease, Inject-Aid, Injection Safety Guard, Insulin Aid, Insulin Needle Guide, and Vial Center Aid. The Novolinpen also has clickers available to help in calculating the insulin dose.

The last chapter of this book will discuss the insulin-delivery machines currently being tested. Until there is a prevention or cure for diabetes, advances continue to be made in both the medications being used and the methods by which they are delivered.

Chapter 7

What Is Important About Exercise?

Exercise has great importance as part of the medical management of the person who has diabetes mellitus. The best exercise program is one in which aerobic activity is done for a period of twenty to thirty minutes on a daily or every-other-day basis.

Benefits of Exercise

There are many benefits of exercise, and they far outweigh the risks. Some of these benefits are improved heart and breathing actions. A most common benefit recognized is the increase in muscular strength and endurance. There is a buildup of lean body mass and a decrease in body fat. The range of motion and the flexibility of the arms and legs are improved. Triglycerides and cholesterol are lowered. High-density lipoproteins (HDLs; the "good guys") are increased, while low-density lipoproteins (LDLs; the "bad guys") are decreased. Blood-pressure control is improved. Depression is decreased. The pain threshold is increased. Both self-image and self-esteem are improved and, most importantly, a sense of well-being is achieved and enhanced.

There are benefits that are even more specific to diabetes management. Some of these are the increased sensitivity of the cell-receptor site to insulin. This sensitivity is noted as a decline in blood-glucose levels due to the improved use of insulin by the cells. The result is a reduction in the total insulin needed.

As exercise is maintained, there is a prolonged blood-glucose-lowering effect. Extensive short-term exercise may even result in lowered blood-glucose levels over a period of twenty-four to thirty-six hours. Some look at exercise as having a possible effect on the length of beta-cell function, especially for those with Type II diabetes and those with newly diagnosed Type I diabetes mellitus. All of these factors lead, directly and indirectly, to a decreased risk for atherosclerosis (one type of blood vessel/heart disease).

Aerobic exercise can be low, moderate, or severe in intensity. It may be rhythmic, but it must be continuous—that is, while walking at varying rates is fine, walking, then stopping, then walking is *not* aerobic. Exercise must be of a certain duration (a minimum of thirty minutes three times a week, or twenty minutes five to six times a week). The major fuels used for aerobic exercise are glucose and free fatty acids. Good aerobic exercises are swimming, walking, rowing, cycling, and dancing (see Appendixes F and G for information on calorie burning). Cross-country (Nordic) skiing is the most effective of all aerobic exercises. Notice that jogging and other high-impact or "severe" aerobics have *not* been placed on this list. There have been too many risks found with such exercise; for the diabetic in particular, the risks outweigh the benefits. Therefore, walking or other low-impact aerobic exercise is recommended.

For an exercise to be aerobic, the heart rate must be at least 50 percent above the resting heart rate. The ceiling level is 75 to 80 percent. The ideal range is between 50 and 75 percent (various books give different figures. The common target range recommended is from 60 to 80 percent).

To determine your target zone or ideal range, first subtract your age from 220. Then multiply this number by 60 percent (or another number, depending on a recommendation by your physician) to obtain your threshold level (the lower number of the range of beats per minute that you aim for during your exercise period). Multiplying the same number by 75 percent will give you your ceiling level. You should aim to maintain a heart rate in this "ideal" range for twenty to thirty minutes (see Figure 7-1: Target Zone). (To feel your heartbeat, place your second and third fingers on the inner side of your wrist or on your neck about three inches below the end of your ear.)

FIGURE 7-1

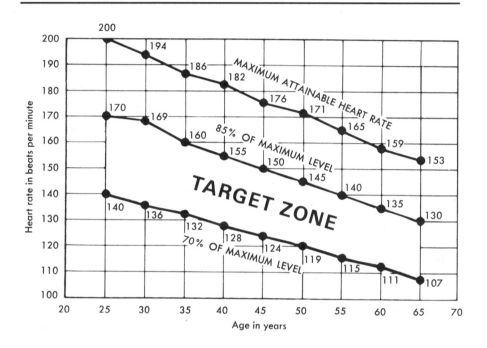

Since you are unable to determine your heart rate every minute unless you have a monitor in place, you can gain a rough estimate of how hard you are exercising by using the "Borg Scale of Perceived Exertion." The scale goes from six to twenty. Less than six would mean sleep or a resting state, while twenty would mean activity to the point of fatigue. Seven would be very, very light activity; nine would be light, and eleven somewhat light. Nineteen is very, very hard; seventeen is very hard; fifteen is hard; and thirteen is somewhat hard. You would try to exercise in the range of twelve to sixteen, or the aerobic-intensity level.

Activities such as weight lifting, gymnastics, and some sports-related activities (e.g., wrestling) are isokinetic exercises. This type of exercise uses glycogen or stored glucose as the major source of fuel. These activities are intermittent, of short duration, and usually quite intense. They are called anaerobic (the person doesn't increase oxygen intake much over usual levels, unlike in aerobic exercise). Anaerobic activities do not offer as much benefit to the person who has diabetes, and in fact they may raise the blood pressure to the point of putting the body at risk.

Precautions in Exercising

Starting any exercise program requires taking some precautions, especially if you have diabetes. First, you must be in the proper shape to exercise. Have your physician evaluate your present condition and recommend any necessary exercise restrictions (such as times or physical states during which you should not exercise). Unless certain heart or eye conditions exist, it is likely that no restrictions will be needed. With blood-glucose testing, you can determine before exercising whether your blood-glucose level is too high or too low to exercise. If your blood-sugar level is less than 60 mg/dl (3 mMol), do not exercise. If the level is greater than 250 mg/dl (14 mMol), check the urine for ketones; if ketones are present, do not exercise. The reason for this is that exercise is a stressor to the body. If the body is "sick"—represented by blood-glucose levels of 250 mg/dl (14 mMol) or greater and by the presence of ketones—exercise would only make the body "sicker" (see Figure 7-2).

Calories need to be adjusted to take exercise into account. The best time to exercise is approximately twenty minutes to one hour after a meal. This allows the food to settle before exercising and gives you the advantage of having some readily available glucose. If the exercise is to be of low intensity or short duration, and the blood sugar is above 100 mg/dl (5–6 mMol), then no extra snack is needed. If the exercise is carried out over a thirty-minute period or longer, then a snack is usually advised (this is more appropriate for high-intensity exercise). For high-intensity exercise, a snack would be eaten beforehand, with another snack eaten every thirty to sixty minutes. Some form of fast-acting simple sugar and an added snack food should be carried at all times. It can be eaten to treat an insulin reaction or to give yourself an

FIGURE 7-2

WARNING SIGNS THAT MAY ACCOMPANY EXERCISE

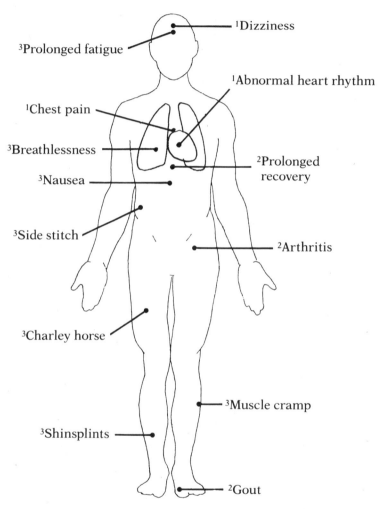

If any of the above occurs:

[1]Discontinue the exercise program.
[2]Try a suggested remedy briefly (such as warmth to the site, or mild gradual stretching to relieve a muscle cramp). If unsuccessful, contact your physician.
[3]You can probably handle it yourself.

energy boost or raise your blood-glucose level after completing the exercise period.

If you have Type II diabetes, and especially if you are also overweight, you do not need to eat extra calories for exercising unless your blood-glucose level drops below normal (the usual between-meal snacks should be continued).

People with Type I diabetes may choose to lower insulin levels rather than increase food intake when they exercise heavily. This would be most appropriate if you desired to lose weight. For a growing child, a teenager, or an active adult, more food (to the level of amounts tolerated) might be the better choice. Some people may not be physically able to eat the number of increased calories needed. Therefore, they might increase calories as well as decrease insulin prior to the time of activity. Such determinations should be made on a one-to-one basis with your health professional.

Before exercising, note the time you last ate or last had an injection. If you are relating the time of exercise to the last injection, then you need to consider the type of insulin, the dosage, the peak and duration of its action, and the site of the injection. Insulin injected into an arm or leg that is used actively during the exercise is bound to be absorbed more rapidly. You would not want to exercise at the peak action time of the insulin without taking special precautions. Note what type of exercise you will be doing and how long you will be doing it.

Be sure that you do not hold your breath during your exercise activities. Also, if you have any eye damage, do not get into a position that places your head lower than your heart. If eye damage exists, don't do any type of exercise that puts strain on your upper body, such as lifting weights.

Exercise with a partner. Teach this person how to treat an insulin reaction so that you have backup protection. Be aware of whether the exercise you are doing is part of your regular routine or if it is over and above what you usually do. Notice whether you are having any pains, aches, or other discomfort. Before you sit down, check to see that your pulse rate is less than 100 beats per minute. Recheck your pulse rate to be sure it is not going above the ceiling level. Be sure you do not exercise when it is too hot or too cold; overheating or becoming chilled can make anyone ill. Wear appropriate clothing (loose cotton clothing, with two pairs of socks and good-fitting shoes).

Any symptoms of insulin reaction mean that you need to stop exercising immediately and treat the insulin reaction. If you do not have *extreme* symptoms (very weak and shaky, with double vision), check the blood-glucose level so that you will learn how much exercise, at what intensity, leads to such a response. Any severe insulin reaction means that you should do no more exercise that day, since the body needs time to recover.

Check your blood sugar about thirty minutes after exercising to be sure that you are not developing hypoglycemia. Eat a small snack if your blood glucose is below 80 mg/dl (4 mMol) after exercising.

Stretching before and after exercising reduces muscle tightness. You must be relaxed when you stretch; if you are not, you can do more harm than good. You should stretch slowly and in a sustained manner. Ten to thirty seconds is the recommended time for the stretching of each of the arms and legs. As you stretch, your breathing should be slow, even, and rhythmic. The major precaution to take is to be sure not to bounce on a stretch, but instead to sustain the stretch for the recommended number of seconds. Be sure that you stretch each part of the body equally.

One more caveat: If your eyes have been treated by laser, you need to be careful in the choice of exercises you do for physical fitness. Exercise should not be done in a position that places the eyes below the level of the heart. If the head is placed lower than the heart in an exercise, there will be an increase in blood pressure. An example of such an exercise would be touching your toes.

The "Exercise Prescription"

The exercise prescription involves four things: the activity you choose, the frequency with which you participate in it, the intensity of your participation, and the duration of the activity. These choices are based on your physical fitness, as determined by your physician. For the frequency, determine whether you are going to exercise three, four, or more times a week. Aim for a minimum of four times per week. Do not allow more than two days in a row to pass without taking some opportunity to exercise. Start slowly—every other day is recommended. Then add more days as tolerated.

The intensity is determined by your target heart rate (the pulse rate above the threshold and below the ceiling). If you are able to sing or talk while you are exercising, then you can assume you are exercising at the proper intensity. Remember the Borg Scale of Perceived Exertion? What is the range of your perceived exertion scale?

The older you are, the more slowly you should start the activity. Even starting with as short a time as three minutes (or, for the very elderly, just one minute) is wise. Gradually increase the time until you reach a goal of twenty to thirty minutes. If your goal is to reduce body fat, you must exercise for forty minutes or longer. Determine what you can tolerate, then add anywhere from one to five minutes each week until you have reached your goal.

Since there are many types of activity to choose from, you don't need to do the same type of exercise every day. Whatever exercise you choose for a given day, be sure it is done continuously and rhythmically (that is, at the same rate or at varying speeds but without completely stopping), that it involves large muscle groups, and that it is enjoyable! If you are bored with the exercise, do some other type of exercise. Boredom may become an obstacle leading to inactivity. On the other hand, don't overload yourself with activities to the point at which you become burned out.

Focus on your goals of cardiovascular endurance, muscular strength, flexibility, and improved diabetes control—and be sure to have fun in the process.

Chapter 8

What About Hygiene?

Daily care is one way to prevent sources of infection that lead to the increase of blood-glucose levels in the body. Daily care involves a number of practices. This chapter will focus on the practices of daily hygiene. These practices involve dental care, skin care, foot care, eye care, and care related to sexually related activities.

Dental Care

Numerous people have reported that once they had healed from having an abscessed tooth, or their gingivitis (gum disease) had been cured, or they had a large cavity filled, their blood sugar became more normal. Any source of infection will "push" the blood sugar up. Therefore, keeping the teeth clean, massaging the gums, fighting plaque, and seeing your dentist every six months or as directed will aid in controlling your blood-glucose levels.

First, you need to know what is recommended for good dental care. People with diabetes, especially older people, should see the dentist more frequently than every six months. If a person has dentures, observations should be made for any inflammation of the gums, with any such inflammation reported to the dentist. Teeth should be brushed or, at least, the mouth should be rinsed after every meal or snack. The major times to brush your teeth are on awakening and before going to sleep. Before going to bed, flossing is a must. Brushing reaches only three sides of the tooth, but the tooth has five sides. Flossing reaches those other two sides. Gum massage is also of help. This could be done with a water pick or with a rubber tip. Placing this tip under the gum line stimulates the flow of circulating blood and assists in ridding the mouth of debris that might have worked beneath the gum line. Flossing usually catches this, but sometimes it doesn't. (Note: To be most helpful, flossing must include the base of the tooth and the area under the gum line.)

If you have a problem with plaque, prerinsing with a plaque-loosening solution is recommended. Many toothpastes also contain ingredients to fight plaque, tartar, or both. The mechanical action of the toothbrush is your best ally in fighting plaque and massaging the gums. The old "from the top of the tooth down" technique has been replaced with the circular or round movement of the brush at the gum line and over the tooth surface.

If any dental surgery is to be performed, blood-glucose levels should be as normal as possible beforehand. The outcome will be better healing at a more normal rate. Antibiotics may be started a few days before the surgical procedure to better support the prevention of infection.

The "quiet occurrence" of gingivitis should also be noted. If you notice any bleeding when you brush your teeth (and you are brushing normally), suspect gingivitis. Severe gingivitis can lead to loosening or loss of teeth and, if it goes under the gum line, bone involvement. Proper dental care and good nutrition, along with normal blood-glucose levels, are the best methods of preventing gingivitis (see Table 8-1).

Skin Care

Skin care is most associated with the simple act of bathing. Surprisingly, there can be both too much and too little use of water. Soaking the body can lead to tissue breakdown, while lack of cleanliness can lead to local infections. Drink plenty of water unless told to do otherwise.

TABLE 8-1

STEPS IN DENTAL CARE

1. Brush teeth at least twice a day with circular, scrubbing motions.
2. Floss teeth at least once a day, making sure to get into the gum line.
3. If plaque is a problem for you, use a plaque-loosening solution before brushing.
4. See your dentist every six months or as directed.

Poor blood-glucose control may increase or reveal such conditions as *necrobiosis lipoidica diabeticorum,* a skin condition that looks much like scar tissue. Individuals with this problem often note that the scarred areas look more "angry" when their blood-glucose levels are higher. Other skin conditions associated with diabetes are also easier to notice with higher blood sugars. For example, xanthoma—a skin condition in which what looks like yellow pimples appear on the skin—may appear. When these pimples are seen, elevated lipid levels (fat levels) are found in the blood. Lowering the blood-glucose levels causes a noticeable lowering of the lipid levels.

If there are frequent boils, carbuncles, or localized infections, high blood sugar and poor skin care should be noted. The sites should be cultured so that the appropriate medication may be given. Until the infections are under control, it is possible that there will be a greater need for insulin.

The need for more insulin may also be true for a yeast infection called candidiasis. Candidiasis may be found in the mouth, under the arms, under fatty folds of the skin, and in genital areas. Local and general medication (medication taken by mouth) may be prescribed. This infection occurs less frequently with lowered blood-glucose levels. If blood-glucose levels are not monitored, the person should suspect high blood-glucose levels the majority of the time if such conditions are noted.

When the blood-glucose levels are controlled, there is less chance that such skin and mouth conditions will occur. If diabetes control is accompanied with good skin hygiene, with bathing done on a daily or every-other-day basis, skin infections should be minimal or nonexistent. (Note: Older people in particular may have difficulty with dry skin conditions if bathing is frequent during the drier winter months.)

Foot Care

Using powders when the skin is moist and lotions when it is dry are general instructions for skin care, and they are particularly important when it comes to the feet. Good care of the feet is necessary to prevent the breaking down of skin areas, since such areas could become sites for infection (see Table 8-2).

The feet are a most vulnerable part of the body when it comes to injury or infection. Walking barefoot and having a lack of feeling set the feet up for some serious problems. If circulation to the feet is poor, the blood flow is not adequate to meet the needs of the healing process. Poor circulation also leads to a lack of healthy nerves. Less-than-adequate circulation may be due directly or indirectly to high blood-glucose levels, which can affect

TABLE 8-2

STEPS IN FOOT CARE

1. Inspect feet daily.
2. Wash feet daily.
3. Dry between toes.
4. Use powder (when damp) and lotion (when dry) and rub in place.
5. Wear clean socks daily.
6. Keep feet warm by wearing warm socks.
7. Cut toenails as directed.
8. Use a buffing pad on calluses after bathing.
9. See a podiatrist for stubborn corns and calluses.
10. Have your physician or other health professional examine your feet four times per year to check the pulse, temperature, and color in order to determine whether your circulation is adequate. You will also be tested for reflexes, vibratory sense, and responses to sharp and dull objects (or just the ability to feel an object touch the foot).

---

the major blood vessels or the cells that act as "insulation" around the nerves. When this insulation is no longer present, the nerves short-circuit (just like two uninsulated wires), and the result is pain, numbness, or both.

Care of the feet is easier for some than for others. An overweight person may have difficulty seeing the bottoms of the feet. Careful and daily assessment of the feet is one of the major ways to prevent problems and to ensure that any problems noted are reported early. You should observe your feet for signs of infection (reddened or swollen areas, pus, a red streak up the leg, pain [if the nerves are functioning adequately]); for corns and, especially, calluses (which can hide tissue breakdown, as this may start under the surface of the callus); for nails that are too long and need trimming; and for areas experiencing pressure (which may indicate that your shoes are ill fitting). Toenails may be sites for fungal infections, which seem worse when blood-glucose levels are elevated. Some people may need help in inspecting their feet.

Besides the sole, an area of the foot that is often missed is the area between the toes. This warm, moist place may harbor infection or breakdown of tissue. Athlete's foot is also most commonly found here.

Cleanliness of the feet is the next thing to emphasize. If the feet are injured, it stands to reason that the possibility of infection will be less if they are clean.

Seeing a podiatrist (foot doctor) for foot problems such as calluses or corns is next in the sequence of care. Calluses that have become enlarged should be filed by a podiatrist. Corn development should be prevented, but if corns do occur you should see a podiatrist. (Note: Ill-fitting shoes may be the problem; daily changes of shoes and checking for pressure areas from the shoes worn are helpful). "Young" calluses or corns can be rubbed, loosened, or removed after a bath.

Toenail-cutting guidelines are as follows: The toenail should be cut following the line of the toe. This is usually stated as "Cut the nails straight across." The curving of the cut into the edges of the toe is not recommended unless the person has problems with ingrown toenails. Ingrown toenails can best be treated by a podiatrist.

Other things to consider are the shoes you choose to wear.

Shoes should be made of leather (so they will breathe), and they should be well fitting. They should be broken in slowly (that is, worn for a few hours the first day, a few more the next day, and so on, until there are no noticeable pressure areas and no discomfort). As noted before, shoes should be changed every day or every other day, whenever possible. Socks should be clean and fit the foot properly. Any creases or wrinkles may prove to be a pressure site after the shoe is in place. Feet should be kept warm with warm socks rather than with heating pads or hot-water bottles.

If you are bedridden, exercises for the feet will be helpful in maintaining good circulation to the feet. These exercises should involve elevation and lowering of the feet, and activity of the feet involving circular and up-and-down movements. Walking is also good exercise for the feet, but only if the shoes worn are well fitting and have good support around the ankles and arches. Walking barefoot is not considered a good thing to do (whether the person has diabetes or not), since there is just too much of a chance that the feet will be injured.

Some people do not consider checking the insides of their shoes for any foreign objects before putting them on. However, sensation may be lost in the foot, and repeated pressure or other injury of the foot—such as that caused by a tack stuck in the bottom of the shoe, or a small toy or other object in the shoe—may lead to problems without the person's really knowing this has happened.

If an injury, such as a cut or scratch, should occur, any alcohol-based product will just burn the tissues and impede (or slow) the healing process. Soap and water works best, followed by careful drying (especially between the toes).

To review: Feet should be washed daily. The water in which they are washed should be warm, not hot. The feet should be dried completely. If the skin is dry, lotion should be applied; if sweaty, powder should be used (be sure the powder or lotion is rubbed in well if used between the toes). After the daily washing, while the skin is still softened, callused areas should be buffed to aid in removing the dead skin, and toenails should be cut as directed. If feet need to be warmed, this can be accomplished by putting on warm socks. Going barefoot is discouraged. Feet should be inspected daily. If problems are noted (for example, infections or pressure areas), you should contact a podiatrist or other health professional.

There is a saying that if you treat your feet right, they will treat you right. This is especially true when you have diabetes.

Eye Care

Eye care is also a part of hygiene. Many illnesses, such as colds and flu, are passed by contact of the hands with either the mouth or the eyes. You should wash your hands before you do anything related to the eyes. If you wear contact lenses, be sure to wash your hands before handling the lenses to prevent eye infections. Any eye infection should be treated promptly. Pinkeye (an acute, highly contagious type of conjunctivitis) can result in blindness if not treated correctly.

For the person who does not have diabetes, routine eye exams should be done every two years. For the person with diabetes, the eyes should be checked every year or even more frequently, as recommended by the ophthalmologist or retinologist. Note: Because optometrists used to be trained primarily to fit glasses, in the past people with diabetes mellitus were advised to see an ophthalmologist or retinologist instead. The reasoning for this guidance was the potential for eye disease with elevated blood-glucose levels. However, optometrists are now educated to look for eye diseases and even to take retinal photographs to look for diabetes-related eye diseases. If a disease is found, the optometrist will refer you to an ophthalmologist or retinologist for treatment.

It is recommended that anyone given a diagnosis of Type II diabetes have an eye exam immediately, with retinal photographs taken. The person who is newly diagnosed with Type I diabetes should have retinal photographs taken after five years of diagnosis. However, it would be wise to have such eye evaluations right away to determine a baseline to be used for later comparison.

Eye exercises are another consideration for good eye care. While this area is somewhat controversial, many people feel that exercises that involve the eye muscles can strengthen the eyes. For example, when you are doing close work, every fifteen to twenty minutes look into the distance and alternate with looking up close, ten times.

Eyes are a very precious part of the body. Your vision can be stable and can last a lifetime if your eyes are well cared for. If treatment is needed, it should be administered as early as possible.

Sexually Related Hygiene

Human sexuality involves the sensual feelings, the reproductive process, gender identification, general cleanliness, prevention of infections in the genital area, and sexual behavior. The genital area can be a source of infection, which can cause blood-glucose elevation. Also, if a person does not feel he or she is functioning well enough sexually, blood-glucose elevation can occur. Pregnancy (which will be discussed in chapter 10 under the heading of "Intermediate Complications") is also a cause of higher blood-glucose levels. Finally, confusion in gender identification may result in stress, which is associated with elevation of blood glucose.

A person's mental health can be affected if he or she becomes worried about diabetes-related problems of decreased sexual functioning. Rest assured that this dysfunction or inability to have an erection or orgasm is probably more mental than physical. If you read some information and suspect you may be having such dysfunction, you are likely to focus on performance rather than enjoyment; this focus will then affect your functioning. If you find that your focus is changed to your performance, get some assistance from a therapist accredited by the American Association of Sex Educators, Counselors, and Therapists. If you still have some questions, speak with your health professional. There are specific tests that can aid in determining whether your sexually associated problems are psychological or physical in origin. Most of the time, you will find that no physical problem exists.

Where physical problems do exist, much can now be done with prostheses (silastic implants that are permanently rigid, semirigid, or inflatable) or assistive devices (such as a vacuum pump and a Velcro belt to place at the base of the erect penis [see Figure 8-1] or the use of papaverine injections), or with hormone therapy.

FIGURE 8-1

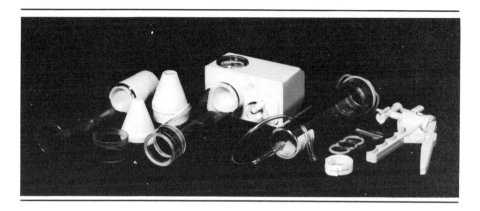

If a problem is suspected and you feel uncomfortable in bringing up the subject of sexual discomfort (some women may feel discomfort with intercourse from having a dry vaginal area due to hyperglycemia or to aging) or performance, write it down and present the problem in written form. If you discuss such problems, you will find that the information will be handled confidentially, as any other body function would be discussed. If other health professionals or students are in the room, ask to speak to the doctor privately. Describe what you think is happening. Your health professional knows what questions to ask to assist you in finding the best solution for the problem, if one is found to exist.

For any treatment, the health professional will take into account your own beliefs and attitudes, your physical developmental history, and whether you see yourself in the male or female role. He or she can either assist you in making changes or offer an appropriate referral.

Your participation in all hygiene measures and your early reporting of any infection or injury will help the health team to keep you in the best possible physical condition. The result will be that you will feel better about yourself and about your health.

Chapter 9

How Is Diabetes Monitored?

Diabetes is known to cause high blood-glucose levels, but how do you know to what extent this has occurred for you? When insulin is too low and glucose levels are too high, glucose is not getting into the cells. How do you know to what extent glucose has not entered the cell and, therefore, to what extent you need another source of energy (fatty acids)? Testing for blood-glucose levels and for ketones in the urine is the short-term answer. For the longer-term answer, testing is done for fructosamine or glycosylated serum protein (such tests show control over the last seven to ten days). A glycosylated-hemoglobin test—especially hemoglobin A_{1c}—provides the longest-term answer, showing control over a period of two to three months by indicating the percent of glucose (attached to the protein in red blood) that is above normal.

Without such testing, people with diabetes cannot know whether their diabetes is really controlled. Regular testing allows you to know the ongoing status of the disease. Keeping blood-sugar (glucose) levels as normal as possible is the best way to prevent or delay vascular (blood-vessel) or neurological (nerve) complications. High blood-sugar (glucose) levels lead to damage of the body cells. It is known that if animals have a blood-sugar level of 150 mg/dl (8 mMol) or more, they develop blood-vessel, kidney, nerve, and eye diseases. It is also known that Pima Indians with diabetes who participated in one study, and who maintained a blood-sugar (glucose) level of 165 mg/dl (9 mMol) or higher, developed these same complications of the disease. The conclusion reached by these and many other studies is that the higher the blood sugar is allowed to be, the greater the possibility of physical problems. Unless blood-sugar levels are controlled most of the time, partial efforts are of little value.

Frequency of Testing

Studies in various parts of the country have indicated that the single blood-glucose measurement, done in the physician's office every few weeks or months, is still the most common method of diabetes management in the United States. However, other studies have demonstrated the futility of this type of management, and more and more people are being treated by physicians who weigh the results of self-testing of blood glucose (SMBG) and glycosylated hemoglobin of some form (such as HgA_{1c} or HgA_1), rather than having a single blood-glucose measurement done.

The philosophy of obtaining a fasting or postmeal blood-glucose measurement in the doctor's office is that blood glucose is relatively stable and that the measurement obtained thus reflects the level over the past few weeks and predicts the level for the next few weeks. Nothing could be further from the truth. We reviewed a patient's chart recently and found the following office blood sugars at three-month intervals: 217, 67, 197, 46, and 125 mg/dl. If management is based on these measurements, the medicine would have been increased at blood sugars of 217 and 197, decreased at 67 and 46, and kept the same at 125. In actual fact, in comparison with the HgA_{1c} the blood-sugar (glucose) averages obtained through self-testing were about the same for each visit, indicating that there was no need for any change in the diabetes medication. Blood sugar is constantly changing, so a blood-sugar test in the doctor's office measures the blood sugar *only for that moment in time.*

The frequency of testing is different for different clinics. Researchers have shown that the more testing done (and responded to), the better the control and the fewer the complications. Lower blood-glucose levels are found before each meal and at bedtime. Higher blood sugars are found after meals. One hour after a meal, the blood sugar would be higher than two hours after a meal. If a person could remember to test for blood-sugar levels on arising and two hours after a meal, more information for control would be obtained than if the more easily remembered premeal and bedtime blood-sugar tests are used. (Table 9-1 lists the steps in testing for blood sugar.) Again, physician preference may guide the person into testing one way or another—that is, testing after fasting and two hours after each meal, or before meals and at bedtime. If the physician does not ask you to do blood-sugar tests at home but does them in the office only, be suspicious that you are not receiving the best of care.

What to Test

Certainly, the blood sugar should be tested if the person feels unusual or ill. Besides the regular testing practices (a minimum of three to four times a day, three days a week for those with Type I diabetes; a minimum of four times a day, one day a week for those with Type II diabetes), other tests should be added as needed. (Remember, it has been found that the more information you get from more frequent testing, the better you are able to use that information to control your blood sugar.)

TABLE 9-1

INSTRUCTIONS FOR TESTING BLOOD SUGAR

1. Wash hands.
2. Pierce finger and obtain "hanging" drop of blood.
3. Start timer.
4. Place blood on strip.
5. Wipe or blot, if indicated.
6. Place strip in machine, if not done at earlier step.
7. Read results at end of test time.
8. Record results.

If blood-sugar test results are 250 mg/dl (14 mMol) or greater, most health professionals would advise that you test the urine for ketones (see Table 9-2). If you are ill, they would usually advise that you test for ketones in the urine *even if* your blood-sugar levels are not high. If you are preparing to exercise and find blood-sugar levels of 250 mg/dl (14 mMol) or greater, you should test for ketones to determine whether or not you should exercise.

Urine testing for glucose is seldom recommended anymore. The major reason is that an elevated or lowered renal threshold will give false information. The renal threshold can be determined by emptying the bladder and testing this urine with the taking of a concurrent blood-sugar (glucose) test. You should then eat a meal, testing the urine and blood sugar one hour, two hours, and three hours afterward. The renal threshold is determined by matching each blood-sugar result with the urine test that *follows* it (not the urine test taken at the same time as the blood-sugar test). The normal renal threshold is at blood-sugar levels of 160–180 mg/dl (9–10 mMol). Children often run renal thresholds of less than 160 mg/dl (9 mMol). Elderly people have a tendency to have renal thresholds greater than 180 mg/dl (10 mMol), and often greater than 200 mg/dl (11 mMol). Remember that damage to blood vessels and nerves begins at blood-sugar levels above 150 mg/dl (8 mMol), so a person with a renal threshold of 200 mg/dl (11 mMol) could have a negative urine test for sugar (glucose) and still be developing complications.

TABLE 9-2

INSTRUCTIONS FOR TESTING URINE FOR KETONES

1. Collect urine in a nonwaxed cup.
2. Dip stick* or strip in urine, or drop one drop of urine on tablet. (If checking for glucose with Clinitest, one tablet goes into the test tube containing either two drops of urine to ten drops of water or five drops of urine to ten drops of water, depending on the "card" you have.)
3. Wait for time requested.
4. Read.
5. Record.

*Sticks or strips may be held in the stream of urine, but be sure the timing is correct.

If blood-glucose tests are unacceptable and the renal-threshold level is known, information from urine glucose tests is helpful. Certainly, such information is better than no information at all. Note that a value obtained from a second passing of urine will measure sugar more nearly representative of what is found in the blood at that time. The first voided test lets the person know what sugar has accumulated over a period of time and therefore provides a better measure over time. Many times, the second voided urine will contain the same amount of sugar as the first urine specimen (such as 33 percent). (For children staying on the "spilling side" of negative, use the two-drop Clinitest method, related to normal or near-normal glycosylated hemoglobin tests in our patient population.) While urine testing for sugar has limited value, it is useful for small children who have tender fingers or for those individuals who have normal renal thresholds. Urine testing for sugar is of practically no value in adults, especially in the elderly.

This brings us back to blood-sugar (glucose) testing. The glycosylated hemoglobin test gives the best overall, average determinations of blood-sugar levels for the longest period of time. The hemoglobin A_1 test (upper limits of normals are around 8 to 9 percent) includes the components or parts of A_{1a}, A_{1b}, and A_{1c}. It is found to respond better to more recent increases or decreases in blood-sugar levels than does the more stable component of this test, the hemoglobin A_{1c} (upper level of normals are around 6 to 7 percent).

There are problems with these tests, however. They can be influenced by sickle-cell disease and other abnormalities of hemoglobin (thalassemia, fetal hemoglobin) and by abnormally high or low hematocrits (the low hematocrit reading will result in a falsely high glycosylated hemoglobin A_{1c}; a high hematocrit reading will result in a falsely low glycosylated hemoglobin A_{1c} reading). If home blood-sugar tests over the past two to three months do not seem to match the results of the glycosylated hemoglobin A_{1c}, then be concerned that something else may be occurring (for example, problems with the machine, with the method or accuracy of the testing, or with hemoglobin or hematocrit levels). Most health professionals prefer to check the hemoglobin A_{1c} every three to six months.

As noted earlier, fructosamine and glycosylated-serum protein levels demonstrate average blood-sugar levels over the past seven to ten days. The first test measures the glucose levels associated with the albumin in the blood; the second measures the glycosylation that has occurred in the other proteins found in the serum of the blood. The second test is more stable than the first, but it is also more expensive. The upper limit of normal for the fructosamine test is 2.8 percent, and for glycosylated protein it is about 8 percent.

Daily self-testing of blood-sugar levels gives the most information. These tests can demonstrate a pattern that may be a reflection of food and medication and of the interactions of these with the person's activity and stressors at home or work. There is a concern about immediately responding to a test result with an increase or decrease of insulin. For a small child, unless he or she is ill, predicting the activity after the extra dose has been given can send the child diving into an insulin reaction. Withholding a dose of insulin because the blood-sugar test is in the normal range may start a series of events leading to a roller-coaster type of response (or to what is termed "rainbow therapy" by some, meaning that you are always chasing the pot of gold at the end of the rainbow but never catching it!). The algorithm method of insulin adjustment is at least based on the giving of insulin over and above the usual baseline daily dose. The person is thus not left with the situation of receiving no insulin and then having to play "catch-up" at a later time.

Unless the person is ill, when supplemental insulin is used to respond to high blood-sugar levels in order to keep the person out of diabetic ketoacidosis, infrequent blood-sugar "spikes" may represent one-time emotional responses and therefore do not require an immediate response. If a pattern develops in the elevation or lowering of blood-sugar levels, something should be done before that blood-sugar response occurs rather than after the fact. Using this approach, health professionals teach people to review their records every two to three days and make adjustments to affect patterns that are observed. Those professionals who use the algorithm approach individualize the amount of insulin to be given when the blood-sugar levels are 150 mg/dl (8 mMol) or higher. If this extra insulin is needed frequently, it is added to the previous dose. For the adult, a combination of both of these methods may be successful.

Using Information from Testing

Perhaps clearer explanations of management methods are needed. There are several methods of managing insulin, as follows:

Method 1: Complete Management by the Physician

The physician may or may not have the patient do self-blood-sugar monitoring. Whatever the testing methods used, all data are brought to the physician, who makes all decisions on changes in insulin and food.

Method 2: Sliding Scale

With this method the patient is allowed to make decisions on daily changes in insulin based on elaborate tables of blood-sugar values and insulin needs. The sliding scale has two major defects. First, insulin is given after the fact—that is, a blood-sugar level at noon, for example, does not predict the insulin needed for the next six hours, but rather reflects the insulin needed six hours ago. You are thus always six hours behind and on a roller coaster of control. The other defect is that there is a cutoff point of blood sugar below which no insulin is given. It must be remembered that Regular insulin lasts only six hours, so even when there is a low blood-sugar level, some insulin must be given to cover the time when the previous dose has run out.

Method 3: Algorithms

Algorithms are formulas for changing insulin. They are similar to the sliding scale, except that the formulas are superimposed on a background of two or more doses of intermediate (NPH or Lente) or long-acting (PZI or Ultralente) insulin. Regular insulin at mealtimes and/or in the evening is changed on a formula basis, depending on the blood sugar at the time. The major defect of this system is that insulin is again after the fact. The system can be made to work, however, by choosing the amount of supplemental insulin based on changes in the food intake or activity levels, or on the consistent need to add extra insulin to the previous dose.

An example of the latter management is as follows: Suppose a person is taking a mixture of NPH and Regular for breakfast, with Regular for supper and NPH at bedtime (a common regimen), and he or she has persistently high blood-sugar levels before breakfast. This person has an algorithm to increase the morning Regular insulin by one unit for every 50 mg that the blood sugar is elevated over 150 mg/dl (8 mMol), and would thus increase the morning Regular if this elevated blood sugar occurred. However, the problem of the increased fasting blood sugar means there is a need for more NPH at bedtime, not for more Regular insulin in the morning. An increase in morning Regular may cause a reaction later in the day. If the algorithm is used, the extra Regular insulin given in the morning should be called supplemental insulin and recorded in the logbook separately.

If the problem is recurrent (several days in a row), then the "supplement" should be added by increasing the evening NPH rather than by taking the Regular continually as a morning supplement.

Method 4: Patterned Glucose Rise

In this method, a basic two-, three-, or four-dose insulin regimen is prescribed, and blood sugar is tested four times (either fasting and two hours after each meal, or premeal and at bedtime) for three consecutive days. The pattern of blood-sugar values is then analyzed, and the appropriate insulin or insulins are altered prior to the time of altered blood-sugar levels. Example: the person is taking NPH/Regular before breakfast, Regular before supper, and NPH at bedtime. The blood sugar is tested after breakfast or pre-lunch, after lunch or pre-supper, after supper or bedtime, and before breakfast. A target range of blood-sugar values for each time period is prescribed, and the achieved values over the three-day period are compared with the target.

If the pre-breakfast blood-sugar level is too high or too low (our target is 60–120 mg/dl [3–7 mMol]), the NPH given at bedtime is changed. If the level after breakfast or pre-lunch is outside the target range (70–150 mg/dl [4–8 mMol]) then the morning Regular is changed. If the afternoon blood sugar is off (70–150 mg/dl [4–8 mMol]), then the morning NPH is changed. If the evening blood sugar is off (70–150 mg/dl [4–8 mMol]), then the supper Regular insulin is changed.

If a different insulin regimen is used, the same principles apply—just remember that Regular insulin acts during the six hours after it is given and peaks in two to four hours; NPH or Lente acts during the twelve hours after it is given, with the peak action time at about six to eight hours after injection. By understanding when a given insulin peaks and what its duration is, you can know when to check your blood sugar and how to use the results to change the insulin dose. Excellent control can be achieved in this way.

Testing Supplies and Equipment

A number of supplies are needed for home self-testing of blood-sugar levels: lancets to pierce the finger, the finger-piercing device, and the machine and/or sticks or tablets used to test blood or urine. The most effective way to clean the fingers is by washing the hands with soap and warm water. Traveling? Alcohol or other cleansing wipes are useful to have.

Urine Tests

Tests for urine ketones are the tablet test, Acetest, and the stick tests (Chemstrip uK and Ketostix). Chemstrip and Ketostix are combined to test for sugar in the urine as well (Chemstrip uGK and Ketodiastix). Glucose-testing strips are also available separately (Chemstrip uG and Diastix). Clinistix, Tes-Tape, and Clinitest (tablets) are also available to test for glucose in the urine. Biotel is available for various screening tests, as are Multi-chem strips.

Lancets

Lancets should be sharp and easy to hold (by hand or by machine). Some lancets fit only some machines but not others. B-D Micro-Fine lancets are made for use with the B-D Autolance. Monoject, Surelet, EZ-lets, and Trends lancets fit most leading devices. The Monoject lancet has a tribeveled point, while the Unilet-Lite and Trends lancets have a beveled edge, supposedly for better penetration with less discomfort. EasyStick and Soft Touch lancets can be used with most units except B-D Autolance and Glucolet. The Sugar System lancet is used with both the Autolet and Glucolet. ExacTech lancet device uses the Ultra TLC.

Lancing machines to hold the lancets are varied. The pen-shaped devices are the Monoject, Pen-let, Soft Touch, ExacTech, Dialet, Hypolet, and Glucolet. The B-D Autolance has specially designed twenty-three-gauge M-D Micro-Fine lancets. The Autolet and, most recently, the Autolet Lite have platforms that control the depth of penetration (see Figures 9-1 and 9-2).

Continual upgrading and improvements have been done on both the sticks and the machines for measuring blood-sugar levels. The quality of these instruments and sticks continues to be high, and technology is improving almost daily.

Sticks

Some sticks are specific for sight reading, while other sticks may be used only with machines or with a combination of sight and machines. The TrendStrips read from 0 to 800 (a two-minute test; three minutes if the blood-sugar amount is over 240 mg/dl [13 mMol]). The Ultra reads from 0 to 600 (a ninety-second test). The Chemstrip bG (timing the same as the TrendStrips), Gluco-stix Reagent Strips, and Diascan Strips read from 20 to 800. When visibly read, Diascan and Glucostix are wiped or blotted after thirty seconds, and TrendStrips require a sixty-second wait before wiping. After an additional sixty seconds (ninety seconds for Glucostix and TrendStrips), the Diascan is read. All the other strips are read by machine (e.g., Glucofilm is used by Glucometer 3). Chemstrip bG has a visual strip reader called the Match-Maker.

Machines

Machines are becoming easier to use (One Touch, ExacTech, Dia-scan S), smaller (Tracer II, the pen-sized ExacTech [now called Medisense], or the credit-card-shaped ExacTech, Glucometer 3), more accurate, and less expensive. There are also new tech-nologies, such as laser and others, which might employ a reusable membrane rather than a disposable strip. There are more sophisticated electronics, such as in the ExacTech, which

FIGURE 9-1

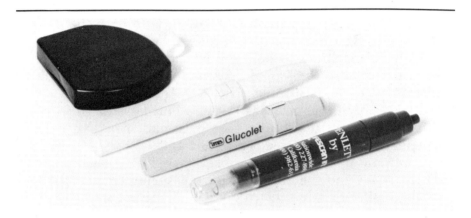

FIGURE 9-2

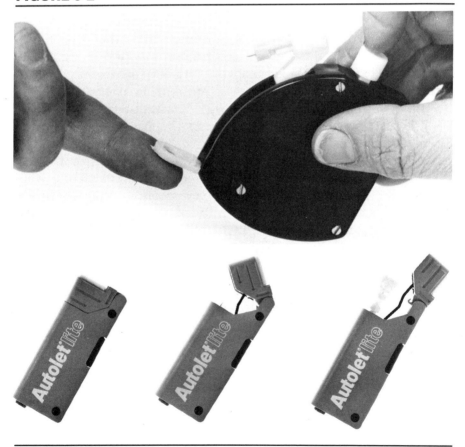

uses an electrical signal rather than a color chemical channel in the strip. AccuChek IIM can now have a "voice" that audibly states the blood sugar, and it is computer adaptable through its electronic logbook, "Merlin" (see Figure 9-3). The GlucoScan 3000 and Lifesan One Touch also have a Memory Bank Data Log system and a display and printout called the Data Manager. Checkmate GlucoScan 3000 (see Figure 9-4), one of the newer machines, has a finger-piercing device built into the machine.

The earliest audio-capable machine was the BetaScan Audio. Diascan-SVM and the One Touch, Touch 'n' Talk package also have audio capabilities. Diascan-S and the Accu-Chek III can notify the user if there is an error in technique. The Glucometer 2 is becoming more refined (i.e., the Glucometer 3 is also now available). The Glucometer 2, Glucometer 3, Glucometer M+, Diascans, GlucoScan 3000, Romeo, and the Trends Meter have memory. Each of these machines holds in its memory a specific number of blood sugars (see Figure 9-5). With the Glucofacts program the data of the Glucometer M can be analyzed by computer and printed for easy access. The Ultra requires no blotting, wiping, or washing. ExacTech, Romeo (Juliet): the DIVA system, Glucometer 3 (see Figure 9-6), Glucofacts, One Touch, Tracer, and Ultra (see Figure 9-7), represent the newest technologies. There are also new technologies being developed that will not have to pierce the skin to give blood sugar.

The DIVA system, the most sophisticated system currently available, uses a meter that can store nearly 3,000 events (such as blood sugar, insulin dose, food intake, and exercise and so forth).

FIGURE 9-3

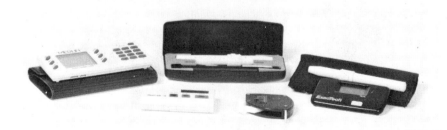

FIGURE 9-4

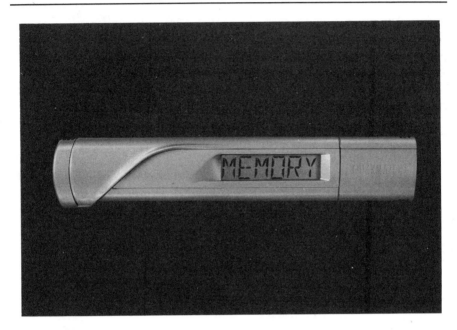

FIGURE 9-5

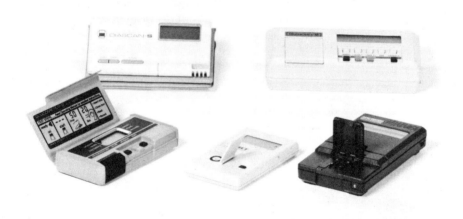

FIGURE 9-6

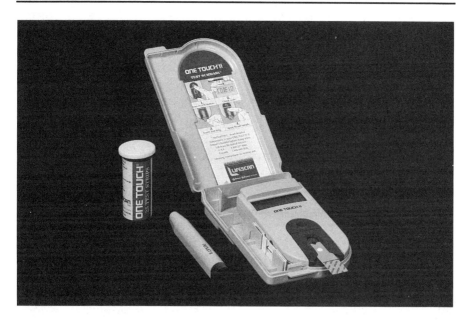

FIGURE 9-7

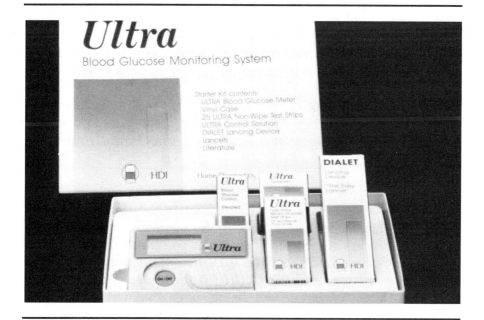

The meter is called Romeo. A desktop dedicated computer called Juliet can analyze the data in Romeo and can even transmit the data through a computer modem to a physician's office computer, which would contain a program called Homer. The system is excellent but very expensive.

Testing is a necessary part of monitoring daily care (see Appendix H for the names and addresses of the companies that make such supplies). Choosing products carefully makes daily care easier. Product quality has proved to be stable throughout the spectrum of those on the market. Any product that has been found to be not up to standard has been immediately recalled by the company for correction.

The most frequently asked question is which machine is best to use at home. All of them are good, so the decision of which one to use should be based on ease of use, readability, cost, and service. Ease of use and service appear to have made it to the top of the list, even over cost. Sometimes people are willing to pay a little more if the service is there. An example of good service is a company's responding to a phone call from you by sending you a machine to use if yours needs to be sent in for repair.

As soon as this book goes to press, new machines will likely become available. Machines will become even easier to use, lighter, and less expensive. One of these days, there will be a machine that does not require the person using it to do any finger sticking. Wishful thinking? Not necessarily. Such a machine is being developed today. And although it will be a while before such machines can be made small enough or inexpensive enough for home use, remember that computers that today can fit in your pocket used to take up the space of whole rooms and cost a fortune. Bloodless sugar testing *will* be a reality in the future.

Summary

Self-testing of blood sugar, the greatest innovation in diabetes care in the last fifteen years, now allows us to attain the degree of control necessary to prevent the serious complications of the disease. Every person with diabetes mellitus, whether Type I or Type II, should be doing self-testing. When diabetes is unstable (such as in illness) or when changes are being made, the testing should be carried out four times per day, every day. When diabetes mellitus is stable, less testing is necessary but is still encouraged.

We feel, from extensive experience, that it is necessary for persons with Type I diabetes to do self-testing of blood sugar (called **SMBG**, for "self-monitoring of blood-glucose") four times a day for a minimum of three days per week. For persons with Type II diabetes, it is necessary to monitor three or four times per day, at least two days per week. For persons taking insulin, whether they have Type I or Type II, it is necessary to have a machine with which to do SMBG. For persons with Type II who are using diet alone or diet plus oral agents, testing with a visual strip is permissible, but machine testing is encouraged.

The data obtained from self-monitoring of blood glucose allow frequent responses through adjustments in the food, diabetes medication, and activity. Combined with frequent measurements by the physician of hemoglobin A_{1c} (Hgb AC), fructosamine, or glycosylated proteins, self-testing is extremely effective in facilitating or permitting good control.

It bears repeating: with good control you will feel better and be more energetic and more productive. Most important, you will be in control of your own life and destiny and will therefore be better able to prevent both acute and chronic complications of the disease.

Chapter 10

Possible Complications of Diabetes

Any time the body chemistry is out of balance, there are bound to be adverse changes in body tissue. The environment, the things you eat, the stresses you are under, and whatever illnesses or disabilities you may be fighting all make a difference in the physiology of your body (that is, the way your body responds). If you have a way to control the "stimulators" of these changes it will be possible for you to minimize the damage that such changes can cause. So it is with diabetes mellitus. The body cells are used to only so much glucose in the system. If there is too much or too little, changes take place in cell function, size, and structure.

There are three series of changes that occur with the person who has diabetes: acute changes, intermediate changes, and chronic changes. Acute changes, or complications, are diabetic ketoacidosis, hypoglycemia, and hyperglycemic hyperosmolar nonketotic syndrome. Intermediate changes are those involving illness, surgery, pregnancy, and travel. Chronic changes are changes involving the nerves (neuropathy), the kidneys (nephropathy), the eyes (retinopathy), and the large blood vessels (macroangiopathy). Chronic changes are noticeable by pain, numbness, inability to see, inability to go to the

96

bathroom, and so on. Retinopathy, nephropathy, and perhaps neuropathy have some association, directly or indirectly, with small blood vessels.

Acute Complications

Diabetic Ketoacidosis

Diabetic ketoacidosis may be preceded by diabetic ketosis, which itself may be preceded by hyperglycemia. As already discussed, hyperglycemia can occur when there is an absolute lack or relative unavailability of insulin. Diabetic ketosis occurs when insulin is deficient and glucose is no longer able to get into the cells, so an alternate source of energy (fat) is needed. The result is ketone production. Diabetic ketoacidosis, the most severe state, occurs when an imbalance due to a severe or prolonged insulin deficiency leads to dehydration and a chemical (electrolyte) imbalance. (See Table 10-1 for signs and symptoms of diabetic ketoacidosis.)

Diabetic ketoacidosis is a serious condition. The blood-glucose levels are not necessarily high (for example, in one case we saw a value of 190 mg/dl [10.6 mMol]). Usually, however, the level is high, in the range of 300–900 mg/dl (18–50 mMol). The production of ketones from the fat breakdown makes the body more acidic. This is when the problems occur, since the body cannot exist if it is too acid or too alkaline. Acidity is manifest or noted by chemistry (biochemically) and by labored breathing (Kussmaul, or heavy and labored, respirations). Kussmaul respiration is the body's attempt to break down and blow off some of the acid in the system (carbon dioxide and its earlier form, carbonic acid).

Diabetic ketoacidosis is treated with intravenous fluids (to dilute the glucose levels in the system and rehydrate the dehydrated person), with insulin (to aid in helping glucose to get into the cells), and with chemicals called electrolytes. Two of the most common chemicals needing replacement are potassium and sodium. These are involved in cellular functions related to electrical changes in the body, particularly in the heart and the brain. The first fluids given are called "plasma expanders," which can be anything from blood to saline. Normal saline (body-balanced salt-and-water solution) is usually the fluid of choice.

Once the blood-glucose levels drop to a certain point (that is, about 300 mg/dl [17 mMol]), the body needs some fuel so that it will not call on more ketones (ketogenesis) and will not drop

TABLE 10-1

DIABETIC KETOACIDOSIS FROM HYPERGLYCEMIA

	SIGNS AND SYMPTOMS	CAUSES	TREATMENT
Hyperglycemia	Increased thirst	Not enough insulin, too much food, not enough exercise, stress, medications	Fluids, insulin
↓	Increased urination		
↓			
↓			
↓			
← **Glucosuria** ↓	Dehydration	Growth, pregnancy, illness	Fluids, insulin
	Blurry vision		
↓ **Ketosis** ↓	Fruity breath		Fluids, insulin
↓ ↓	Weight loss		
↓ ↓	Acetone in urine		
↓ ↓	Blood sugars usually over 250 mg (14 mMol)		
↓ **Ketoacidosis** ↓	Electrolyte imbalance		Fluids, insulin, potassium, other chemicals as needed
↓ ↓	Nausea		
↓ ↓	Vomiting		
↓ ↓	Kussmaul respiration		
↓ ↓	Pulse fast and "thready" (i.e., thin, weak)		
↓ **Coma**			
→ **Hyperosmolar Nonketotic Syndrome (seldom seen in Type I Diabetes)**			Fluids, insulin, potassium, other chemicals as needed

---

below normal blood-glucose levels (hypoglycemia). Glucose is then added as part of the saline solution (D5 or D10 usually in half of normal saline). The choice depends on whether there is a balance in the saline level in the body, as determined (analyzed) by frequent electrolyte determinations in the lab. Potassium is almost always added to the intravenous fluids, as are other chemicals, if such chemicals do not return to normal in the rehydration process. Insulin is also given, usually intravenously, until the blood-glucose levels are near normal and stable.

Hypoglycemia

Hypoglycemia can be separated into the true low-blood-glucose state or the "false" state that mimics low blood glucose. The adrenaline that is released when the body feels that it is in crisis causes the symptoms of shakiness, trembling, irritability, hunger, and weakness that are usually associated with perceived hypoglycemia.

"False" hypoglycemia occurs when the blood-glucose level is still in the normal range but drops rapidly over a short period of time, or when it reaches a level to which the body is unaccustomed. If the person has had very high blood-glucose levels for a long period of time and values drop rapidly, symptoms of hypoglycemia may occur. To date, the literature demonstrates only that if the blood-glucose levels drop 50 mg/dl rapidly, the symptoms do not occur. Symptoms are usually experienced when the blood-glucose levels fall faster and/or in greater amounts (that is, 100 mg/dl [6 mMol]). The symptoms are those of adrenaline release, not of true below-normal glucose levels or of hypoglycemia (see Table 10-2 for signs and symptoms of hypoglycemia).

True hypoglycemia occurs when blood-glucose levels fall below the normal range of the test (that is, 60 mg/dl [3 mMol] for whole blood). Hunger, some irritability, and perhaps a little weakness occur when the levels are 40–60 mg/dl (2–3 mMol) (Level I). At 20–40 mg/dl (1–2 mMol) (Level II), dilated pupils, trembling sweating, and a stronger, more rapid pulse rate occur (remember, this type of pulse rate indicates only that adrenaline has been released and so can also occur with false hypoglycemia). Unconsciousness, seizurelike activity, or other neurological manifestations are seen when blood-glucose levels are below 20 mg/dl (1 mMol) (Level III).

TABLE 10-2

INSULIN REACTION—HYPOGLYCEMIA, INSULIN SHOCK

SYMPTOMS		TREATMENT
Mild:	Irritable, trembly, weak, shaky, hungry	Food (general snack—carbohydrate and protein)*
	Blood sugar 41–60 mg/dl (2–3 mMol)	Food or drink (one-half to one calorie point in milk, or a snack with protein and carbohydrate). Next regular meal or snack as scheduled, then rest for 15 minutes. Contact a health professional.
Moderate:	Skin cold and clammy to the touch; pale face; shallow, fast breathing; drowsy	Simple sugar (20–40 calories); small snack 10–15 minutes later; then 15 minutes of rest.
	Blood sugar 21–40 mg/dl (1–2 mMol)	
Severe:	Unconscious, possible convulsions, danger of swallowing incorrectly	Glucagon injection; simple sugar; food with protein 15–20 minutes later.
	Protect person by placing on side or stomach, and keep airway open.	Notify physician.
	Blood sugar usually less than 20 mg/dl (1 mMol)	

WEAR MEDIC ALERT BRACELET!

CAUSES OF INSULIN REACTION

Unusual physical exertion or exercise without increasing food or decreasing insulin

An overdose of insulin or pills due to a mistake in measuring

Mistake in the meal plan

Failure to reduce insulin after an infection

Poor usage of the meal due to vomiting or diarrhea

Delay in eating a meal or snack

*Important note: If blood sugars are low at injection time, be sure to treat until the blood sugar is up to 100 mg/dl (5.5 mMol), then take injection and have something to eat immediately.

Symptoms are different from person to person. If a person has had Type I diabetes over a long period of time (that is, five years or longer), it is possible that the symptoms may change. Some specialists feel that in such a case the body has become overchallenged over the years. Whatever stimulated the release of adrenaline before is now ignored, and the body therefore loses its warning system.

As noted earlier in this book, food in small amounts is often all that is needed for Level I hypoglycemia. Level II usually requires some simple sugar to bring the blood-glucose level up to 40 mg/dl (2 mMol) or to relieve symptoms. Food will usually be used properly at blood-glucose levels greater than 40 mg/dl (2 mMol).

Level III requires 50 percent glucose, glucagon (see Figure 10-1), or some thick liquid glucose product (for example, honey), placed either in the cheek or under the tongue. If a person is having seizurelike activity, it would not be safe to give oral sugar, since it could be inhaled into the lungs. At home, injection of glucagon into muscle tissue is the preferred treatment. (Note: if glucagon is used, simple sugars are given to replace glycogen stores and to overcome nausea when the person arouses; food can be given after the person is no longer nauseated.) Every insulin-taking person with diabetes should have glucagon available at all times—at home, at school, or when traveling. (Note: Dosages for glucagon are ¼ mg for three years of age or younger; ½ mg for four- to five-year-olds; 1 mg for anyone older than five.)

Hyperglycemic Hyperosmolar Nonketotic Syndrome

This syndrome is a subtle but quite severe hyperglycemic episode in which the acid does not develop but dehydration is very acute. (This condition is called a syndrome rather than coma, because the majority of these people are diagnosed before they ever reach the state of coma.) Blood-glucose levels may be in the neighborhood of 800–2,000 mg/dl (44–110 mMol). *Osmolarity* is the level of water concentration, or dehydration, of the body. The higher it is, the worse the outcome for the person involved. Dehydration must be attended to first; insulin is then given in carefully prescribed doses, as individuals with this condition are very insulin sensitive.

FIGURE 10-1

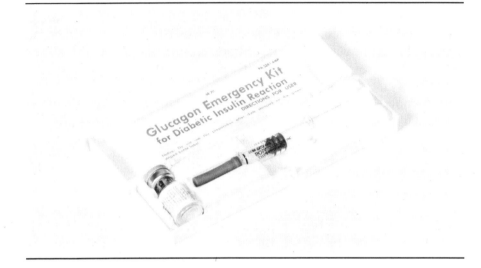

In diabetic ketoacidosis there are ketones in the blood and urine. In hyperglycemic hyperosmolar nonketotic syndrome, there are few, if any, ketones in the blood and urine, because the person is making just enough insulin to suppress ketogenesis (the making of new ketones). The large amount of fluid lost also means the loss of much potassium. Replacement of potassium is done during the acute state and usually for some time afterward. The more potassium lost and the greater the state of dehydration, the more seriously ill the person.

Intermediate Complications

Intermediate complications are those that involve various stressors such as illness, emotional upset, surgery, pregnancy, and travel.

Complications Due to Illness and Stress

More insulin is required during most illnesses. A few illnesses, such as those with vomiting and diarrhea, require either less insulin or a delay in insulin administration. The usual response to high fever is higher blood-glucose levels. The more ill or dehydrated the person becomes, the higher the blood-glucose levels will be. The object in dealing with the illness is to keep the diabetes out of the picture (i.e., the illness acts as a stressor that could cause the person to go into diabetic ketoacidosis. If the diabetes is adequately treated, then only the illness needs to be treated). If the medication taken is in a sugar solution or in some other way elevates blood-glucose levels, the insulin may be raised. If the person is on an oral agent or on diet alone, insulin may be required during the acute phase of the illness.

Prevention is, of course, best (for example, getting flu shots and keeping immunizations up to date). If an illness does occur, vigorous treatment is needed. If the illness or treatment causes the blood-glucose levels to go up, increased insulin is needed. (Note: Prolonged emotional stress will act just like an illness on the body, so treatment needs to be the same. The higher the blood-glucose levels, the more insulin is needed, depending on ketone levels.)

Whether you have Type I or Type II diabetes, it is important during illness or stress to monitor your blood-glucose levels carefully and frequently. Your health-care team should have given you some rules for what to eat and drink at these times and how to supplement your insulin doses or alter your oral agent. To make these changes in medication, however, you need to know your blood-glucose values. If you have these data, it is a simple matter of mathematics to respond appropriately and prevent diabetic ketoacidosis or hyperglycemic hyperosmolar nonketotic syndrome.

Complications Due to Surgery

Surgery, whether for a minor or a major problem, is also a stressor to the body. If the person is on an oral agent, the physician may request that the agent be discontinued for from one day (for short-acting oral agents) to three days (long-acting) before the surgery. Insulin may then be used during surgery for the person with Type II diabetes.

If the person has Type I diabetes, normalization of blood-glucose levels prior to, during, and after surgery will help the healing process. If the blood-glucose levels are elevated, there is a decrease in fibroblasts (the cells that heal wounds) and white blood cells, with the result being a greater chance of infection. (Note: If scientists want germs to grow on an agar plate, they add one thing—glucose.) Many specialists are recognizing that some insulin is needed. It may be given in a smaller amount without food, or in a somewhat larger amount when the intravenous fluids are begun in preparation for the surgical procedure.

Complications with Pregnancy

If the blood-glucose levels are kept normal from prepregnancy through delivery, the chances of having a normal baby are the same for a diabetic woman as they are for a nondiabetic woman. If the blood-glucose levels are not controlled during the first trimester of pregnancy (the first three months), there is a 14 percent chance of congenital problems, fetal loss, or maternal complications. The goal is to maintain the blood-glucose levels in the range of 60–90 mg/dl (3–5 mMol) fasting, and 70–120 mg/dl (4–7 mMol) two hours after a meal. This is true for women with gestational diabetes (diabetes just during pregnancy) as well as for women with Type I or Type II diabetes. If a woman has been on oral agents, she must be started on insulin during pregnancy because of the potential side effects of oral agents on the fetus. If a pregnant woman has more difficulty in controlling blood-glucose levels, insulin is given via an infusion pump or in four or more doses of short-acting insulin per day.

Complications During Travel

Much preplanning must be done so that travel, whether for pleasure or for business, is a safe and rewarding experience. If you are going overseas, a company called Diabetes Traveler (P.O. Box 8223, Stamford, CT 06905) can give you the names of doctors in other countries who know about diabetes management. As noted earlier in the book, this company can also tell you what supplies are available in what countries and how to ask for assistance in other languages.

   If you will be crossing more than one time zone, many specialists advise you to change to multiple doses of short-acting insulin, which may be given just before meals (usually every four hours on an overseas flight). An insulin-infusion pump or baseline insulin (Ultralente or PZI) make it even easier to travel. You need only to take insulin in bolus or injection before a meal, whenever it occurs. It is usually recommended that you stay on multiple doses for twenty-four to forty-eight hours after you reach your destination. The two cardinal rules for travel: Always keep your insulin with you (not in your suitcase), and always keep some food in your possession.

Chronic Complications

Chronic complications are perhaps the most feared, even though when they are caught early there is a chance of reversing some of the processes. It is only when there is an end-stage process working (that is, when there has been cell damage or destruction) that little can be done. Again: The best way to prevent or delay complications is to keep the blood-glucose levels in the normal range as much of the time as possible.

Neuropathy

Neuropathy is easily recognized by burning and tingling sensations, pain or numbness, and lack of function. The pain associated with neuropathy often decreases with lowered and normalized blood-glucose levels, but it may even increase temporarily. The discomfort of neuropathy may be worse at night, and you may feel some discomfort from the bedclothes touching your feet (an object can be placed on the bed, with the covers placed over it so that they do not touch your feet). No one knows just why the discomfort increases. Perhaps as new blood vessels form and as the nerves become resensitized or new ones grow, they become more sensitive. The increased discomfort may thus mean that something is improving rather than that something is wrong. Your physician will assist you so that you can be as comfortable as possible during this uncomfortable time (the discomfort usually lasts from about six months to a year).

Some people feel more discomfort with exercise, even just mild walking. This discomfort may not be related to neuropathy alone. Pain in the legs with walking that is relieved by rest is probably caused by an obstruction to blood flow in an artery of the leg due to diabetes or general vascular (blood vessel) disease (that is, you can have high cholesterol levels but not have diabetes). This cramping condition is called "intermittent claudication." A medication may be given that allows the blood to flow more freely through the blood vessels. Another treatment is to open an artery through angioplasty (a balloon) or laser treatment, or through surgically bypassing the obstruction (bypass graft).

Numbness is the other side of the coin. As noted in an earlier chapter, people have experienced bizarre episodes such as having a tack in the foot without knowing it until they do their daily foot inspection! This is why daily foot inspection is so important (along with not going barefoot).

There are five different types of neuropathy, as follows (see Table 10-3):

TABLE 10-3

DIABETES NEUROPATHIES

Polyneuropathy (reversible)	Disease of the end of the nerve	Sensory loss or weakness of hands and feet; absent reflex
Autonomic Neuropathy (treatable, but not as easily reversed)	Disease of part of the nervous system that controls automatic body function (such as the heart, glands, or intestines)	Gastropathy (disease of the stomach—also called gastroparesis), sexual dysfunction, diabetic diarrhea, lack of sweating or increased sweating, stopping of heart or of breathing, postural hypotension (i.e., feeling lightheaded when quickly changing from a lying to a sitting or standing position)
Diabetic Amyotrophy (reversible)	Disease of the end of the nerve	Weakness and loss of nerves to muscles in hands, thighs, and pelvic area
Mononeuropathy (reversible)	Disease of spine and cranial (head) nerves	Pain, weakness, sensory loss, or change in reflexes
Radiculopathy (reversible)	Disease of beginnings (roots) of spinal nerves	Pain or sensory loss in an area of the skin

DISTAL SYMMETRICAL POLYNEUROPATHY   This type, also called simply polyneuropathy, involves the feet and legs and is usually described by the person as numbness or tingling in the feet. Sometimes a burning sensation is noted. Normalizing blood-glucose levels is the best treatment at present.

AUTONOMIC NEUROPATHY   This type involves nerves that work without your needing to pay any attention to them—for example, nerves relating to control of the blood pressure (orthostatic hypertension), to the stomach or gastrointestinal tract (possible problems include disease of the stomach [called gastroparesis] or the intestine [diabetic diarrhea]), the sweat glands (loss of the ability to perspire), to the bladder (problems with urinating), to balance, and to sexual function. Autonomic neuropathy is not as closely associated with diabetes control as is peripheral neuropathy (neuropathy of the hands and feet), but diabetes control is still needed. There are a variety of other treatments that can control the results of autonomic neuropathy.

PROXIMAL MOTOR NEUROPATHY   This type involves damage to the nerves in the muscle, resulting in weakness (also called diabetic amyotrophy) and shrinking of the muscle fibers. A burning sensation may also be experienced. The hands and thighs are most commonly affected, and the ankle joint may also be involved. Resolution or recovery may be experienced in from six to eighteen months.

CRANIAL MONONEUROPATHY   This type of neuropathy most often involves the eye muscles. Double vision may be present; the eyelids may droop, and the eyes may drain. Mononeuropathy may also involve the spine. Improvement in either of these is usually seen in three to four months.

RADICULOPATHY   This type begins at the roots of the spinal nerves. Pain or sensory loss may be experienced on any part of the skin surface.

Recently, there has been documentation of improvement in the various forms of neuropathy with normalization of blood-glucose levels. This has given added support to the need to keep blood-glucose values under 150 mg/dl (8 mMol) for prevention of problems and for reversal of changes that may have already occurred.

Microangiopathy

Small-blood-vessel disease (microangiopathy) is responsible for many problems related to the kidneys (nephropathy), to the eyes (retinopathy), and to some degree to the muscle of the heart (cardiomyopathy). (While heart disease is associated mainly with macroangiopathy, some microangiopathy also occurs.)

KIDNEY DAMAGE (NEPHROPATHY) Nephropathy may be associated with infection of the kidneys, ureters, bladder, or urethra. Infection of the urinary tract is common in people with diabetes because of sugar in the urine and/or because urine may be kept in the bladder as a result of neuropathy. If the infection starts in the bladder and either occurs over and over again or goes up the ureters to the kidneys, damage to the kidneys may occur. Any damage to the kidneys will eventually result in decreased kidney function. Diabetic nephropathy (damage of the kidney) is often a result of blood-vessel damage, with scarring of the filtration system of the major part of the kidney. This may be caused by thickening (and thus weakening) of membranes in the blood-vessel walls as a result of elevated blood-glucose levels. Bleeding could occur, or protein could leak from these blood vessels.

Checking for protein in the urine helps in early detection of renal disease (note, however, that protein in the urine is not always due to kidney damage but can also be due to some other stressor, such as infection or intense exercise). Control of hypertension is extremely important, as is prompt treatment of any urinary-tract infection.

Where kidney damage has occurred, renal dialysis (washing the blood out through the use of a machine) or, as a last resort, renal transplant now offer hope of improved quality and quantity of life. Improved tissue-matching techniques and new immunosuppression drugs (medicine to keep the recipient from rejecting the transplant) have resulted in more successful transplantation.

RETINOPATHY Retinopathy may occur in various stages, the earliest of which are more reversible. Stage I involves the formation of a microaneurysm, which is the ballooning of a weak wall of a blood vessel. Microaneurysms may burst and hemorrhage. Exudates, or defined yellow spots, can sometimes be seen. While these were once thought to be fat or lipid deposits, they have actually been found to be scars from areas of bleeding in the retina. Stage II involves new vessel formation, hemorrhage, and scarring. Once this has occurred, it is not possible to reverse the condition. However, stabilization is possible through laser treatment.

The lens of the eye may also have problems. In the presence of higher glucose levels, the lens can become more translucent than transparent, and osmotic changes (the pulling of fluid into the lens) can result in a cataract. This leads to blurring of vision. The cataract can be easily removed and a new lens transplanted.

If hemorrhage (bleeding) has occurred in the eye, the fluid in the eye may become cloudy. Removal and replacement of this fluid may restore clear vision and can also help to remove scar-like membranes that have formed on the retina.

If there is too much pull on the retina, as can occur because of multiple bleeding episodes and subsequent scarring, the retina may pull away from the back wall of the eye. Retinal detachment can be corrected.

Retinopathy need not inevitably cause blindness. When retinopathy is discovered early and treated vigorously, vision can be preserved.

Macroangiopathy

Large-blood-vessel disease most often affects the heart, but it may also affect the brain or the extremities. Heart attack, angina (pain), and coronary disease are related to damage to large blood vessels. The blood vessels feeding the heart can become obstructed, resulting in death of part of the heart muscle, causing a heart attack. In the brain, a rupture or blockage of a blood vessel could occur. Because part of the brain would thus not be receiving adequate nourishment, unconsciousness or paralysis results. New treatments can help greatly in recovery from these occurrences, especially heart attacks.

If the blockage involves the extremities, disease affecting the arms and legs (peripheral vascular disease) can occur. Intermittent claudication (cramping pain on walking due to partial blockage of the blood vessels, as discussed earlier) is associated with this type of problem. Hardening of the arteries (arteriosclerosis) can involve any large blood vessel. If the blood can't get through, the loss of the affected part of the body is possible. Any pain or decreased blood flow in the lower extremities should immediately be called to the attention of your physician.

Peripheral vascular disease can be treated with a variety of techniques, including angioplasty, laser treatment, and bypass grafts. The simplest of these is balloon angioplasty, in which a catheter is placed in the artery and fed to the area of blockage. A balloon is then inflated to squeeze the fatty blockage against the vessel wall and open the vessel.

Complications, whether acute, intermediate, or chronic, can usually be controlled. Much is being done to prevent and overcome these problems. Your participation at any stage of development of such a problem will assist you in achieving better, or at least more stable, health. It is important that you keep yourself aware of any changes in your body, as well as of changes in treatments that might be of help to you.

Over the last ten years, the Diabetes Control and Complications Trial investigators tested and observed 1441 people who were divided into study groups. There were two major groups: insulin dependent people who had no signs of complications of diabetes and an insulin dependent group who had early signs of diabetes retinopathy. These major groups were then sub-divided into groups labeled (see Appendix K for definitions), "Intensive Control" and "Conventional Control." The results of the study, that were reported during the American Diabetes Association's National meeting in June (1993), were the following: in the "Intensive Control" group there was a 76% reduction in the risk of having eye disease (retinopathy), there was a 56% reduction in the risk of having kidney disease (nephropathy), there was a 61% reduction in the risk of having nerve disease (neuropathy), and there was a 35% reduction of the risk of developing a high level of bad cholesterol (LDL). The average hemoglobin A1c was 7.2% in the "Intensive Control" group (8.9% in the "Conventional" group). The down-side was the weight gain and, as the researchers learned more about managing diabetes, a decreasing but over the usual number of severe insulin reactions. The up-side? "Intensive Control" can be achieved, but it requires hard work, a well motivated person with diabetes, and a well trained health care team.

Chapter 11

How Do You Adjust to Having Diabetes?

How do you adjust to the diagnosis of diabetes or to being told that you have one or more of the complications of the disease?

Reacting to the Diagnosis

If you have just received the diagnosis of diabetes, or if you have just heard of someone else with diabetes who is suffering from a variety of problems, you may be somewhat fearful. In any case, you know that having this disease will have a significant impact on your life and on your family's life. As our mentor, Dr. Robert L. Jackson, has stated, "This is a disease that has the potential of helping families to grow." As complicated as the management program may seem, Dr. Jackson feels that it can be basically simple: eating nutritious foods to meet the needs of growth and activity levels; taking the amount of medication needed to cover the food and activity; and testing to see whether the decisions have been correct.

When you are first diagnosed, it is not helpful to you when others say that at least it's better than having cancer (or some other disease), however true this may be. Even when they say, "You'll become more healthy because you'll learn how to really take care of yourself," it does not help at first.

111

You're too emotionally involved to be ready to learn at this point. Perhaps you'll even find yourself saying some of these things to others about your diagnosis. Your family and friends may feel awkward around you. You can guide them by telling them that they don't need to say anything; they just need to support you. Simply saying, "I'm sorry this has happened to you" or giving you a hug can be enough at this time. Talking to another person who has had diabetes for a while helps, too (see Appendix I for help in finding a contact near you through your local diabetes chapter of your state affiliate).

Seek out support people: those with whom you can talk comfortably and to whom you can display your true feelings and thoughts.

Ask your family to keep junk food out of the house; to not tempt you by offering you sweets; to give you an injection now and then (if you were really ill, this would come in handy); to learn how to treat an insulin reaction; and—especially for immediate family members—to attend diabetes-education classes with you.

When the emotional edge is less and you start asking questions, then go to a source to learn as much as you can.

If you feel that you really haven't adjusted to the diagnosis of diabetes or to having a complication of the disease, consider some other ways of thinking. Consider the ways of healthy living that are part of your control of diabetes. This knowledge could be shared with others. In the case of a complication, consider being grateful that the complication was discovered at an early stage, if true, or that stabilization of the complication is more possible now than it was ten years ago. Consider talking to a counselor, pastor, or psychologist. There may never be an answer that satisfies you, but once you can accept the reality that you have diabetes or a complication, grasp this as a challenge, then get actively involved. As noted earlier, in some situations early diagnosis of a complication and improvement of diabetes control can reverse or slow the progress of the complication.

The Grief Response

You may feel angry or depressed. These emotional responses are common, and it is *all right* to have—and to recognize—these emotions. People respond in varying ways to news that is not considered pleasant. This response is often termed "the grief response." The grief response includes the emotional responses of denial, anger, bargaining, depression, and acceptance. These may occur in sequence, but some may be experienced at the same time. Allow the grief process to occur. Don't try to be superhuman or stoic. Remember that the grief response is natural, and that it is okay for your family as well as you to have such feelings.

DENIAL.   This is often the initial response to diagnosis. Denial might be expressed as "It's not really true."

ANGER.   This is often expressed as "Why me?" Anger can occur at the same time as denial. The diagnosis might be blamed on a family member, on an accident, or stress at work, or on some other factor.

BARGAINING.   Bargaining involves weighing the odds. Most often, the person denies that choices made today will influence his or her health status later on.

DEPRESSION.   This emotion seems to reappear time and time again, with varying intensity. Depression noted shortly after diagnosis of the disease appears to reach some resolution in six months or so. Reminders of the disease (for example, medical costs, blood-sugar tests, and doctors' appointments) may trigger depressive episodes. The person may even decide not to monitor blood-sugar levels or see the doctor.

ACCEPTANCE.   This is a time of resolution. Denial is no longer present, and the person asks what she or he needs to do to get on with life. Acceptance signifies the person's readiness to learn.

Let's return to discussing depression. This emotional response is often misunderstood. There are two types of depression: pathological and functional. Pathological depression occurs when a person is no longer able to make rational decisions, talks less or stops talking altogether, or withdraws. Surprisingly, this occurs no more or less often in persons with diabetes than in the nondiabetic population. Functional depression is considered less severe and is usually resolved with education and support.

Defense Mechanisms

Anger, denial, and bargaining may be associated with responses called defense mechanisms. The major defense mechanisms are rationalization, regression, reaction formation, repression, withdrawal, and compensation.

Rationalization means saying, for example, that something desired but not obtained was no good, anyway.

Regression, which is more noticeable in adults than in children, means becoming more dependent on other people to cook food, give shots, monitor the disease, make decisions, and so forth. Or, a person may regress by not taking appropriate care of himself or herself.

Reaction formation can be described as a person's doing the opposite of what he or she has been told to do. For example, if told to decrease caloric intake, this person responds by "pigging out."

Repression means that a person "forgets" what he or she is supposed to do, either subconsciously or consciously. An example of repression is a person "forgetting" to take insulin.

Withdrawal represents a more acute sense of depression. A person may feel that all is hopeless and may therefore do nothing at all.

Compensation, which is a positive defense mechanism, means taking a negative or handicap and actually making a positive out of it. The person works harder to overcome something that, by some standards, would be considered an obstacle rather than an opportunity.

Compensation is one way of reframing, or looking at something (such as a statement or action) in a different light. For example, while having a chronic illness is a definite negative, you could look at how healthy you have become through improved self-care routines. With skill, you can take almost any situation or thought and reframe it in a positive way.

Parents of children who have been diagnosed with diabetes commonly report feelings of guilt: "I somehow gave this to my child." Some parents rebel against this feeling by acting out in ways that make the child feel rejected. Through their actions, such parents are stating, "My child is less than perfect. This child is no longer mine." Parents need to recognize that in our present state of knowledge, there is nothing that can be done to prevent a child from developing diabetes.

Self-Esteem

Your self-esteem involves who you think you are, what strengths you feel you have, and what you feel you have achieved. Your level of self-esteem will have a great deal to do with how you react to having diabetes. If you have low self-esteem you may feel over-whelmed, become too dependent, be afraid of change, and even, through poor choices, be self-destructive. Or you might respond in an opposite manner, being too boastful or ignoring other people's feelings. In either case, you need to improve your level of self-esteem.

Your self-esteem can be assessed by considering your mental, emotional, and physical self. This assists you in developing a realistic image of yourself. Once you accept yourself as you are, you can take pride in the things you have done. Your activities and accomplishments assist you in developing self-confidence—a very important part of self-esteem. Recognize that it is all right to fail, and that you have the courage to learn from failure and to go on. You may also have felt guilt. Recognize that guilt is a thing of the past. Use it as a learning experience about yourself, without condemning yourself.

You can improve your self-esteem by developing a knowledge about your good points. Use these good points to assist you in enhancing your self-confidence. Become a friend to yourself. Know that you are a unique being. Choose to risk to allow yourself to grow.

Family Support

There are a number of things you can do to support yourself, and that your family can do to help support you. The first step is to aid your family in recognizing that diabetes is an illness that will not disappear. Get some help for all of you if you or they seem to be dwelling on any part of the grief process. A professional therapist or counselor can support and guide you and your family through the thinking process. Most of all, allow you and your family time. Adjusting to any disturbing news takes time. You may want to think about going to a diabetes camp, either as a camper or a counselor (see Appendix J for the name of the American Diabetes Association camp closest to you). Encourage your family members to learn as much as they can. Help them to know the definitions of diabetes-related terms (see Appendix K). Encourage them to attend chapter meetings of the American Diabetes Association. Both you and they can become support persons for others.

Some people say they have never adjusted to having diabetes. Others, however, say that once they and their family reached the point of acceptance, they chose to fight the disease and its potential consequences with all the weapons available to them. One of the most important weapons is family support. Such people choose to feel that they are controlling their diabetes rather than that the disease is controlling them.

Chapter 12

How Stress Affects Diabetes

Anyone who has diabetes must become aware of anything that encourages the release of glucose into the bloodstream. The result is an elevated blood sugar. This physical response is different in each person, due to individual emotional and physical factors as well as environmental considerations. As already noted, being diagnosed as having diabetes is stressful, as is being told that you have a complication of the disease. Having various pressures in life that influence the control of the disease is also stressful. *Any* event or information could be the "stressor." Any physical response you have to that event or information is called stress. When you experience stress, your body responds by circulating blood faster. Glucose is "poured" from its storage sites (the liver and muscle sites) into the bloodstream. Your blood pressure increases, as does your pulse rate (except in a frustrated type of stress response, in which your pulse rate may actually slow down). A variety of signs and symptoms may be noted, including dilation of the pupils.

Acute Response

The most frequent, rapid response a person experiences during stress is called the alarm (or acute) response. It is termed "acute" because the adrenaline release occurs within a short time. The brain sends a message to the adrenal gland, telling it to secrete adrenaline. This adrenaline release, which may take from seconds to minutes, occurs when the blood glucose is too low, when the person is scared or excited, or when the body thinks it is at risk. When adrenaline is released, there are many physiological responses. Adrenaline stimulates an increase in heart and pulse rate. It is also indirectly responsible for the cooling effect of the body (perspiration). Blood vessels in the hands and feet narrow. For the person with diabetes, the most common responses experienced with hypoglycemia are due to adrenaline release. This adrenaline release results in weakness, shakiness, and a strong, rapid pulse. These symptoms stop when the blood-glucose levels rise to normal. When the sugar in the system is already high, the person usually feels the response of high blood sugar rather than the adrenaline released. The major purpose of adrenaline release in a person with diabetes is the subsequent release of glucose into the bloodstream. It is thus both a blessing and a curse: a blessing in raising low blood sugar, and a curse in adding to the problems of diabetes control by rapidly raising the blood sugar above normal (in the case of brittle diabetes, discussed later in this chapter).

Chronic Response

In most cases, the acute response rebalances the body, making the person able to deal with the problem at hand. The chronic (day-to-day) problems associated with having diabetes affect the body somewhat differently. A little cortisol release is helpful; a lot is not. Cortisol is a steroid type of hormone, released from the outside section of the adrenal gland. The body's response to cortisol is to increase blood pressure and to decrease the pulse rate. Other things that happen are a decrease in the number of white blood cells and the changing of amino acids (protein) into sugar (glucose). The release of these cortisol types of hormones occurs in minutes to hours.

Other hormones in the body that affect the blood-glucose levels, either directly or indirectly, are glucagon, thyroid-stimulating hormone, and growth hormone. Growth hormone is released even in adults; the result is a greater mobilization of fats for energy, leaving glucose in the bloodstream. All of these counterregulatory hormones wreak havoc on blood-sugar control. Even when no food is eaten, blood-sugar levels can be high at one time and low at others. Some doctors have termed this "brittle diabetes." Whether it has to do with lifestyle or with poor management, the results are the same.

Other Responses

Although there are multiple factors that lead to the physical stress response, it has been found that these factors are not as simple as originally described by world-renowned stress researcher Dr. Hans Selye. Multiple causes, which vary from person to person, are responsible for the body's physical, mental, and emotional responses. Dr. Selye's General Adaptation Syndrome can be adapted to assist you in knowing why you feel the way you do when your blood sugar is low, and why your body becomes your own enemy when your blood sugar is high.

The first phase is rightly called the *alarm* phase. The feelings you get could be associated with acute happenings such as diabetic ketoacidosis and hypoglycemia. The feelings are most noticed when you are in hypoglycemia. Blood pressure rises, the pulse rate increases, and you feel shaky, nervous, tense, and anxious. Sugar is made available to the body due to an adrenaline release.

The second phase is that of *resistance*. This is associated with the release of steroid-like hormones. The person has a sense that nothing can be done. If a person diagnosed with diabetes has difficulty adjusting to the disease physically, mentally, and emotionally, self-care may be ignored. The chronic high blood sugars lead to changes in the body cells, which can lead to complications.

The third phase is the *exhaustion* phase. While complications during the other phases are usually reversible, in this phase they are less so. If control is established so that stability is maintained, a little improvement might be noted, but problems are still likely.

However, in individual cases in which there have been some eye, kidney, and neurological changes, some women have chosen to become pregnant once these problems have been contained. With teamwork, a positive outcome of a healthy baby and a stable mother has been shown to be possible. Keeping the blood-glucose levels normal throughout the pregnancy can thus enable a woman to have a good pregnancy despite her body's being in the exhaustion phase of stress due to diabetes.

Stress Management

What can you do about stress? There are a number of ways to handle it. Becoming your own PARENT is one.

Positive Thinking

Believe it or not, you can increase the release of the hormone endorphin, which leads to increased physical strength, if you think positively. If you consider a person you know to be a negative thinker, you may also recognize how frequently that person is ill. Positive thinking is thus associated not only with physical strength but also with an improved level of health.

Attitude

Your attitude comes from the beliefs you have and thus develops from the inside out. Your attitude affects your diabetes by supporting you to make correct choices. Therefore, a good attitude is very important in self-management.

Relaxation

There are many ways to relax. These may be partial relaxation or complete relaxation. It is interesting that after spending much of our lives conditioning ourselves to respond to stress, most of us actually need training to learn how to relax properly. First, you need to become aware of whether what you are currently doing to relax is *really* relaxing to you. Check this out by getting an alcohol thermometer. Hold the bulb lightly between the thumb and forefinger until the red-dyed alcohol is stable, indicating the present body temperature of your hands (this is called "peripheral body temperature"). This temperature indicates how relaxed you are.

When the temperature of your fingers is in the seventies or eighties, it usually means that you are more tense (or cold!). When it is either in the nineties or four degrees higher than your previous temperature, you are more relaxed. The more the peripheral blood vessels open (dilate), the more the muscles have relaxed and the more blood flows unobstructed to your fingertips.

After you have noted this temperature, do what you normally do to relax (for example, read, watch TV, walk, or work on a hobby project). After ten or twenty minutes, sit quietly for about a minute with your hands in your lap, then take your peripheral body temperature again. If you have completely relaxed, this second temperature should be four degrees higher than the first temperature, as noted earlier. If the temperature hasn't changed or is lower than the previous temperature, note that the activity you tested, while not necessarily bad, is not an activity to undertake if you want to relax your body.

The training goal of relaxation is to get into a state in which you "get out of the way of yourself." Any process may be used, but all approaches must have one thing in common: they must focus your mind on something other than your problems. Deep breathing, progressive relaxation, autogenic therapy, meditation, and imaging are some of the techniques that can be used. The training process for any of these techniques will take anywhere from six to ten weeks, with practice periods of ten to twenty minutes, preferably twice a day.

DEEP BREATHING   Two to three deep breaths are taken for immediate release of tension. For deeper relaxation, seven to eight breaths are recommended. This is deep, abdominal breathing, and lightheadedness can occur if you get up too quickly afterward.

PROGRESSIVE RELAXATION   This is a process of contracting and relaxing the muscles, beginning with the toes and moving up to the face. You learn to sense how the muscles feel by contracting the muscles for ten to twenty seconds and sensing how they feel in that contracted state, then relaxing these same muscles and sensing how they feel in the relaxed state.

AUTOGENIC THERAPY   The same muscle sequence can be followed as in progressive relaxation. In this approach, you imagine that your muscles are very heavy (relaxed). When the muscles surrounding the blood vessels are relaxed, these muscles become warmer due to unobstructed blood flow. This is a physical, or mechanical, response rather than an imagined response.

MEDITATION Traditionally, the focus here is a sight or sound. For example, a mantra or other specific sound might be repeated over and over again. Dr. Herbert Benson, associate professor of medicine at Harvard, is a leader in the stress-management field. Dr. Benson has people focus on the repetition of the word *one* as part of his program involving the "relaxation response." Other people use prayer or a scripture. Still others concentrate on a picture or on a spot on the wall. As relaxation ability improves, the relaxation response can occur within a shorter period of time.

IMAGERY This technique takes your focus away from your problems. The imaging can take the shape of people, places, or things, or it can involve focusing on bright to calm colors (and back) or bright to calm music (and back). Visualizing an accomplishment, such as climbing a mountain with supportive aid as needed (from family, friends, or spiritual strength), gives a feeling of accomplishing a goal and the peace and good feelings that accompany it.

Biofeedback

Biofeedback is a technique in which you learn to use information about changes in your body. Relaxation training may be enhanced through biofeedback, such as might be obtained by measuring skin resistance, muscle-energy output, or temperature of the hands or feet. The initial use of biofeedback is just to let you know how you are responding to changes in thought or position. Later on, it aids in training you to become more relaxed by letting you know which types of activities represent your "getting out of the way of yourself" so that your body automatically relaxes. The key is not to *try*. (Remember what happens when you *try* to go to sleep? You are more wide awake. Similarly, if you try to relax, you will become more tense.) Instead, *allow* yourself to become relaxed by focusing your thoughts away from the hectic problems of the day.

Exercise

Exercise is next. Exercise not only helps you to feel good about yourself, but when done on a daily or every-other-day basis it can decrease depression, increase the pain threshold, and improve cardiovascular strength. To be effective as a form of stress management, the exercise must be participated in for twenty to thirty minutes daily or every other day. When you are mentally tired, exercise will act as a stimulant. When you want to be more creative and more organized, exercise will stimulate these attributes. Too much exercise, or exercise performed when the body is in a stressed state (that is, with blood-sugar levels of 250 mg/dl [14 mMol] or greater, or during illness), will only lead to a stressed state or will aggravate the existing stressed state. Exercising wisely can aid in decreasing the physical stress responses of the body. Be sure that food and/or nutrients are timed and are in the proper amounts to give you the best support.

Nutrition

Nutrition is perhaps one of the most important antistressors available. Good nutrition is really very subtle in its actions. Just as with diabetes, outwardly you may not be aware of any difference, but inwardly the body is responding differently. As you become more aware of the impact of nutrition on your body, you will notice changes in skin tone, a sense of alertness, less bloating or other intestinal problems, and so forth. For stress management, you need to think not only about how much you eat but about what you eat, when you eat, and how fast you eat.

As with earlier advice on nutrition, most of the directions for nutrition related to stress management apply to the nondiabetic person as well.

How is nutrition useful as an antistressor? Eating the appropriate amount for the activity or for growth and development is helpful. An overloaded stomach leads to sluggish thinking and sluggish activity. The composition of the food determines the nutritional status of the body. Purposefully planning to replace nutrients that have been used or to take in the right nutrients at the right time leads to better health. Eating at erratic times can throw the body out of balance, not only in terms of the digestive functions but also in terms of the time action of medication taken to control blood-glucose levels. Sweets are empty calories and don't make you feel good. And too much of any one food—whether it is sweets, high fiber, or anything else—can throw your body out of balance and result in some organic effects.

Touch

There are a variety of different definitions for the term *touch*. If you reach out to others, you in turn feel the effect in yourself. Touch also relates to therapeutic massage—that is, the loosening of muscles through touch so that you achieve a relaxed state both physically and mentally. Massage can give relief to tense and stiff muscles and it can increase joint flexibility and range of motion. It aids in reducing blood pressure. It can assist in improving the capacity for clear thinking, and it gives a feeling of well-being.

One technique of therapeutic touch is taught by Dora Kuntz and Dr. Delores Krieger. In a sense, it involves very little actual physical touch but is a process to determine and smooth the energy fields of the body. You could learn to do this to help another person or to teach another person to do it for you when you are in some discomfort. The bibliography at the end of this book includes the name of a book that can help you to understand and learn about this therapy.

Then there is the exhilarating touch of giving or receiving a hug. A hug increases the heart rate and circulation and aids in an all-around feeling of being "okay." June Biermann and Barbara Toohey prescribe four hugs a day. Others have stated that we all need four hugs a day for survival, eight hugs for maintenance, and twelve hugs for growth!

Stress management involves taking responsibility for your own self—for your thoughts and your actions. It means that you may become more mature, that you are able to take the "good news" of self-care and turn it into a level of self-management that leads to a healthier mind and body.

As you learn how to include stress management in your own life and how to relax, you may find that your blood-sugar levels are getting lower and more stable. Keep in touch with your health professional(s), since less medication may be needed.

Chapter 13

Helping Your Health-Care Team to Help You

The total management package for people with diabetes requires a team effort. Like any management package, diabetes management requires all parts to function. Most of all, it requires you to follow directions, think through your program, and have input into that program. Nothing can happen without interaction between you and your physician (and other health-team members). Some of the additional team members are the nurse in the hospital or clinic, the nurse educator, the dietitian, the counselor or psychologist, the social worker, the podiatrist, and the exercise specialist.

Program Management

The physician is the manager of your program. The nurses in the hospital or clinic see that you get the right medication at the right time and that you are monitoring yourself to the best of your ability. The nurse educator works closely with the physician to coordinate resources in the hospital or office and to assist you in carrying out your program. The dietitian makes sure that you know what your food choices are and why and when you should eat certain foods. The counselor or psychologist (or psychiatrist, if medication, psychoanalysis, or neuropsychiatric assistance is needed) is on the team to assist you in your adjustment to having a chronic illness and in thinking through the impact it will have not only on your life but also on the lives of your family and friends. The social worker's job is to assist you in the financial realm and in developing or mobilizing community support. This person might also be involved in some counseling, especially for rehabilitation services, if needed. The podiatrist is included to be sure that one of the most vulnerable areas of your body—your feet—are kept in good condition. The exercise specialist helps you to develop your individual exercise prescription, which includes the type of exercise and its frequency, timing, and intensity.

Other key specialists, if they are needed, might include a cardiologist, a nephrologist, an neurologist, an ophthalmologist (or retinologist), a gastroenterologist, and an orthopedist.

All care must, of course, be kept in balance. To do this, you must test your blood sugar regularly and monitor your food intake, your activity, and your medicine. You must take note of the way you feel and of whether you have had a reaction. You also need to be aware of any other factors that can help you to personalize your program.

The information must be correct and complete. Accurate input from you, even though it may seem embarrassing at times to give this, will allow your physician and other health professionals to design the most useful and safe program to meet your needs.

Record Keeping

To help the health team help you, you should be sure that your records are as accurate and complete as possible (see Table 13-1). These records also act as a teaching tool for you: accurately obtained and kept, such data can give you assurance concerning how food and insulin or other diabetes medication result in changes in your blood-glucose levels.

To best accomplish the feat of record keeping, look to some of the various companies that offer free blood-glucose monitoring booklets, or develop your own on paper or through the use of a computer. Be sure to have your name and some identifying data in place, such as an address or phone number; in case you lose your papers, this information will help in the return of the records.

The next two important items are dates and times. There should be places to record variations in information about certain foods, different times, type of low blood-glucose response, and so on. In recording, the columns should be set up so that you could see a pattern, if one exists. For example, you might find that at 11:45 A.M. every day you have an insulin reaction, or that you have a blood-sugar level greater than 200 at 3:00 every afternoon. This would give you guidance as to the need for a change in food or insulin or an oral hypoglycemia agent prior to that time.

In some programs you will be given guidance, within set limits, to alter your food, medication, or activity prior to the time a pattern occurs. If you saw that each day, at about the same time, you were having a higher blood sugar (e.g., 204 mg/dl [11 mMol]), you would learn to increase insulin, decrease food, or increase activity prior to the time of day the elevated sugar had been noted. The increased number of tests done increases the ability of the physician to help you. It has been shown that the more one conducts tests and then contacts the health professionals or makes educated changes, the more normal the blood-glucose levels are.

In any case, be sure to have at least three days of what we'll call "profiles." A "profile" means performing a minimum of four blood-glucose tests per day at the requested times (for example, *fasting* and *two hours after each meal*, or *premeal* and *bedtime*). These records, along with such other information as the glycosylated hemoglobin test and glycosylated protein or fructosamine levels, will aid in the decision-making process of whether to change or maintain your present program.

One woman who had attended a diabetes education program went in to her appointment with her physician with her well-kept record booklet. Her physician looked briefly at the booklet and then told her that she didn't need to bring in so much information. As the woman was walking out of the office, she saw the physician dropping the record book into a wastebasket. She was so shocked that she turned around, picked up the record book, and promptly changed physicians. The physician probably did not know how to interpret the data, and the woman was wise to find a physician who could interpret the data and support her in achieving good control.

TABLE 13-1

MONITORING RECORD

Name: _____ Phone: _____
Address: _____ City: _____

Date:	Time:	Time:	Time:	Time:	Time:	Comments: Foods, Activities
Blood Sugar / Ketone						

Date:	Time:	Time:	Time:	Time:	Time:	Comments: Foods, Activities
Blood Sugar / Ketone						

Sample:

Date: March 3, 1991	Time: 7 A.M.	Time: 10 A.M.	Time: 2:30 P.M.	Time: 8:30 P.M.	Time: 3:00 A.M.	Comments: Foods, Activities, etc.
Blood Sugar / Ketone	110	94	290 / Neg.	110	(Not Done)	Ate at party at 2:00 P.M.

Reporting

Other ways you can help are by promptly reporting the occurrence of any severe insulin reactions. Most of the time, you will be able to recognize why a severe reaction has occurred. If not, a change in management is needed right away. If a change has occurred in your lifestyle, if you plan to travel (especially for the first time), or if you are experiencing a lot of stress and find that, even though you have followed through with your program, the desired glycemic response is not occurring most of the time, you need to report to your management team so they can assist you in making changes in your program. Tell them the problem, and, as needed, give them the last two to three days of blood-sugar readings and urine ketone results if a blood-sugar reading has been greater than 250 md/dl (14 mMol). Also tell them of any changes in your food intake or activity.

No matter how insignificant a particular piece of information may seem to you, it may be the most helpful in assisting your diabetes team to help you. Remember: (1) test/monitor, (2) record, (3) report.

Chapter 14

Helping Your Family and Friends

Your diagnosis of diabetes mellitus affects not only you, but your family and friends as well. This "ripple effect" is due to the time and energy you need to use to take good care of yourself. While you need support from your family and friends, in time they will need to be supported, too. It goes both ways; with support going each way, the necessary physical and emotional adjustments can become a part of everyday activity.

Increasing Their Understanding

Be sure a family member or friend goes with you when you attend diabetes education classes (as mentioned earlier in this book, when you are questioning what was said, two heads are better than one). In this way, the other person will also have the opportunity to learn what to expect, what is involved, how to treat an insulin reaction, and how to prevent subconscious sabotage of your program. Perhaps this last item is one of the most important. That "one little bite won't hurt you" comment can lead to more bites of food than are desirable for you. If friends or family do either too much for you (smothering you) or too little (ignoring you and your disease), you may feel upset. Both situations are unhealthy for you, mentally and emotionally. You need to be educated to the point at which you become independent in your own self-care. If everything is done for you—your shots, blood-glucose tests, meals, and so forth—then you feel like less of a person. You become more dependent on the other person, and you stop growing. On the other hand, if a family member refuses to discuss your disease and your feelings, shuns your company, or refuses to help you with shots when you are very ill, you will likely feel rejected.

In a healthy, balanced situation, friends and family members support you in self-management. They are willing to give you an injection or blood-glucose test if necessary, and to purchase your supplies when you are ill. Hopefully, you can also share some of your feelings with them without their scolding you or getting upset.

Gaining Their Support

You can help your family in many ways, some of which may be quite subtle. One way is to see that your family receives diabetes education. This gives them some understanding of how they can be of assistance. It also gives them a recognition that they have emotional responses to your disease, too, along with guidance for handling these emotions.

Offering to let family members give you a shot or do a blood-sugar test gives them practice in case you really need their assistance at a future time. It also indicates that you trust them enough to allow them to do these procedures. Some people may have real fears about giving an injection. Encourage them to recognize that insulin is a lifesaving medicine. Indirectly, oral agents are lifesaving also.

If someone is still unable to participate in your care, recognize that you may feel some sense of rejection. Try to assess the situation from the other person's standpoint. On the other hand, if you refuse to let a family member or friend give you a shot or do a blood test, do so with some explanation of your fears. If this is not done, the other person may experience a sense of being rejected. Your family members and friends need to feel that they are accepted and/or that they are a part of your care.

Family meetings can be most helpful. This is a specified weekly period of time (usually from thirty to forty-five minutes) when family members can meet to exchange ideas, discuss feelings, and work on plans. If children are involved, they should be encouraged to take leadership roles. The meetings also help siblings to understand one another (which is especially helpful if it is a child who has diabetes), and to understand themselves. Sibling rivalry is increased if a sibling doesn't know why the child with diabetes is receiving so much attention.

Try to be as realistically independent as you can about the care of your disease. As soon as you are able to do so, give yourself the majority of your injections, and do most of your blood-glucose tests. Learn your meal plan so that you can make appropriate choices from the food that is served (education helps the family to cook more nutritious food, if you are not involved in the grocery shopping and cooking). If you are visiting friends and are offered a food you should not have, you can simply say, "It's not something I am able to eat," or "My doctor hasn't included that on my meal plan," or, with humor, "My doctor would slap my hands if I even aimed a fork in that direction."

Humor is most helpful in your adjustment and in the adjustment of family or friends. When you are able to joke about yourself, others will feel more comfortable in your presence. If you were to walk into a house and state solemnly, "I have diabetes," chances are that your hosts would be walking on eggshells. Your attitude plays a large part in the attitude of others toward you and toward your diabetes. A joking comment in the right place at the right time can make everyone feel more at ease.

Grieving

You, your family, and your close friends will all experience some grief at the time you are first diagnosed or when any complication is diagnosed. Grieving is a normal part of any feeling of loss. Just as it is for you, it is normal for your family and friends to grieve. Just as you might experience disbelief and denial, so might they. When the reality hits that your diagnosis means a change in schedules and meals and makes it necessary to learn new information, family and friends may respond by not saying anything or by nagging you, by walking away from you or by keeping too close. Education and counseling will be useful to them, as perhaps you found such support helpful. They don't need to say anything; they just need to listen.

Chapter 15

What Is Being Done to Conquer Diabetes and Improve Its Management?

Research brings hope to all those who have diabetes mellitus and to their families. If no research were being conducted, one would have the sense that no one cared, that no one felt that there was any hope. Hope is the lifeblood of the person with diabetes. Whether it is today or tomorrow, new findings will improve the life of anyone who has diabetes.

Transplants

You have diabetes, and you want it cured. Today, ideas seem to be focused on the use of either a pancreatic or associated transplant, or the implantation of an artificial pancreas.

Transplantation of cells or body parts from one person to another (for example, beta cells; islets of Langerhans, which contain the beta cells; or partial or complete pancreas) has been attempted over the last 15 years. Drugs that suppress the invasive system of the body (immunosuppression) must be taken once the transplant is in place in order to prevent rejection of the transplant by the body, which recognizes that what has been transplanted is not its own. "Pure" beta cells (that is, those that have no attachment to other tissues) have been found to have the least rejection possibilities. If a person is given just a part of the pancreas of a living person, the results are similar to the transplant of a kidney or heart.

Whole or partial pancreatic transplants are currently being performed in several centers around the world. Although this procedure has improved the diabetes status of recipients, rejection and infection are problems.

Dr. David Sutherland, a world-renowned transplant surgeon, has stated that the most effective and long-lasting transplants are those in which the kidney and the pancreas are transplanted at the same time. In over 300 transplants performed since 1978, there has been a 75 percent success rate for the simultaneous transplants but only a 60 percent success rate for the transplant of the pancreas alone. (No increase is needed in the immuno-suppressant drugs when two organs are transplanted instead of just one.)

Islet-cell transplant research also continues, but at a slow pace due to lack of funds and a government moratorium on the use of fetal tissue in research. No transplants are being done outside a research setting, and few are being done at all in the United States. Animal and laboratory research continues, though at an agonizingly slow pace.

Much research needs to be done in this area. Funding is inadequate, and restrictions are great. Availability is also a problem, whether a partial pancreas, beta cells, or islet cells are involved. Yet transplantation remains a promising area of research and a bright hope for the future.

Artificial Transplants

The artificial pancreas is called a "closed-loop" system because it is self-regulating—that is, it contains all the elements of a real beta cell and can regulate itself in controlling the blood-glucose level. Such a system would consist of a sensor to find the current blood-glucose level, a computer or brain to run the system, a pump to inject the insulin, a reservoir to contain the insulin, and a power source to run the system. Ideally, the system would contain a reservoir of glucose or glucagon to counter low blood sugar. With space-age technology and the miniaturization of computer chips, such a system is becoming more and more possible. The biggest obstacle is finding a machine (a glucose sensor) that, when placed inside the body, would indicate the blood-sugar level and send a message for the need of insulin, glucose, or glucagon. To date, all the materials tried for an internal sensor have been walled off within the body (covered with fibrous, fatty tissue) anywhere from a few weeks to a few months after the device has been implanted. The walled-off sensor does not sense the true blood-glucose level and thus does not give accurate information.

Once this obstacle is overcome, the next obstacle will be installing a "fail-safe" system or component to counter any malfunction. This could be a section of the closed-loop system in which glucagon might be injected. The glucagon release, at a preset blood-glucose level, would aid in raising the blood sugar.

The main part of this newer closed-loop system is already being studied in human subjects. It is about the size of a hockey puck and it contains a reservoir for concentrated insulin. An inside computer, programmed by an outside computer through radio-transmitted signals, directs the release of minute amounts of insulin. The amount of insulin to be released is signaled by the results of the finger-stick blood-sugar test.

An outside closed-loop system called the Biostator can test and control blood-glucose levels. From a catheter in a vein, less than half a teaspoon of blood per hour is heparinized (so it won't clot and block the tubing). This heparinized blood travels into the machine through tubing, past a glucose sensor that signals the machine to give insulin or glucose in a specific amount, based on blood-glucose levels. Although this machine is useful for quick management problems, it requires a highly skilled staff when used for routine purposes (such as during surgery or labor and delivery) or for research purposes.

New Treatments

Insulins are today more refined and much purer than they were in the past. We are now able to make biosynthetic insulin (with pork insulin changed to match human insulin) and biogenetic insulin (growing other cells that make insulin, such as wheat cells or certain cells normally found in the digestive tract). Pure human insulin can be made simply and inexpensively. However, the purer the insulin, the shorter its duration, so there was a trade-off involved in reaching the goal of purity.

Pro-insulin—the chemical before it becomes insulin—was studied in some depth. It was found that pro-insulin has some of the same timed activity as intermediate-acting insulin (such as NPH), and that insulin could be stylized to meet individual needs. Some people absorb short-acting or intermediate-acting insulins at differing rates of speed, and stylized insulin could be developed to meet their needs. These stylized, or "designer," insulins are currently being developed and tested.

As noted earlier in this book, methods of giving insulin are becoming more sophisticated, and these methods will become less expensive and easier to use with further research. One company is now working on a machine that uses a special probe called a transducer, which is placed on the skin. Through the use of certain electronic signals, the machine can be directed to measure the amount of sugar in the tissue fluid and adjusted to read the amount of sugar in the blood. The machine is fairly large and expensive, and at present it is being designed for use only in a physician's office. Once the machine has been thoroughly tested and placed on the market, the company intends to reduce the size (and the price) for home use. The cost of the home machine is expected to be about $2,000 (but note that blood-glucose strips will no longer be needed).

Some exciting new therapies have been developed for Type II diabetes. New oral hypoglycemic agents are being tested, as are combinations of different oral agents and of oral agents and insulin. New dietary treatment is being developed for weight loss and blood-sugar control. There are new findings about the way insulin works and why the body's system goes wrong. Scientists are currently making good progress in learning about Type II diabetes, and we are very optimistic about the future.

If you have an idea for a new diabetes treatment, mention it to your family physician. If it seems in any way possible, contact your diabetes association for the name of a researcher in your area. Write up your idea. If you have difficulty writing, describe it into a tape recorder or in a face-to-face discussion. Get your idea to that researcher. Don't be afraid of being turned down. Perhaps your idea has already been tried. But again, perhaps no one has tried what you have thought up in exactly the same way. If you have the resources, find out ahead of time whether your idea has been tried before. If not, most researchers who know about diabetes will know whether the information you discuss is new or old.

Education for you and for professionals helps to develop new ideas. The American Diabetes Association has developed a set of medical standards to guide health professionals in diabetes management. As they learn about these standards, they may question them or determine that they would be best carried out another way. In other words, the health professionals will stimulate thinking in regard to what is being done, aid in upgrading what is done, and stimulate ideas as to how things can be done better.

The effort to do things better means that there are people who care, and that change is possible for the person who has the disease. Is it best to learn what causes diabetes, how best to manage it, or how to cure it? For those who have the disease, the cure is the focus; for those with a strong family history of diabetes, prevention is the focus. For ongoing care, ways to treat diabetes are the center of attention. Scientists therefore approach diabetes from all of these angles.

Finding the Cause

If diabetes were able to be prevented, then there would be no need for special machines or surgical procedures. Finding the cause would pave the way for prevention of diabetes and is thus extremely important.

The diabetes syndrome, in most of its forms, is basically genetic, or inherited. As noted before, however, it may have many other causes (e.g., it may result from surgery, certain medications, or other stressful diseases). Type II diabetes is an inherited disease, but the gene of inheritance, and even the chromosome that carries it, have not been positively identified. Work continues in several centers to identify the gene, and we are hopeful that it will soon be identified so that someday we may be able to modify it and cure or prevent diabetes mellitus II.

The gene, or genes, for Type I diabetes is closer to being identified. Type I diabetes, which is associated with the study of the immune system (immunology), is a syndrome of diseases rather than one disease. Immunology is closely associated with inherited traits (genetics). People diagnosed with diabetes are often found to have family histories of the disease. Genetic markers are now being revealed, and it someday may be possible for people to take a blood test that will show whether they are predisposed to get one of the diseases of this syndrome. Perhaps some future research will lead to the ability to make changes based on such findings so that a person can avoid both developing the disease and passing it on.

Research is progressing rapidly in determining the relationship of the immune system to Type I diabetes and developing chemicals to stimulate or suppress the immune system. While this work is still in its early stages, we are very hopeful that a way to prevent Type I diabetes will be found in the not too distant future. We strongly hope that this is the last generation of children who will develop Type I diabetes.

The Question About Lispro Insulin

Lispro is a new insulin preparation which, at the time of this writing, is not currently available on the market, but which should be available within the next year. This is one of a group of insulins known as designer insulins since they are designed by computer and then produced. They are the result of manipulation of the amino acid sequences in the insulin molecule. In the case of lispro, it consists of a single alteration in and the insulin molecule simply switching positions for lysine and proline in the terminal end of the B (beta) chain of insulin. In the normal molecule proline comes before lysine and if one simply switches these and puts the lysine first, it changes the properties of the insulin particularly the rate of absorption.

One of the disadvantages of regular insulin is that it takes about 30 minutes or more to be absorbed from the tissue and 2–4 hours to have the peak effect. Since food is absorbed in 1–11 hours, the insulin has to be given 30 minutes ahead of the meal which is inconvenient. Likewise, the duration of action is a little long so that it may produce hypoglycemia prior to the next meal after the food from the previous meal is gone. The lispro is designed to be absorbed much more quickly and can be taken within 5 or 10 minutes of the meal time. It has a very quick peak that corresponds to the absorption of food. It therefore has the convenience of being able to be taken when the individual eats, whenever that may be, and a quick rise to blunt the rise in the post meal blood sugar when the food is absorbed. It then disappears very quickly about 2 hours or so. Thus it does not cause the late pre-meal hypoglycemia so often seen with regular insulin. The one disadvantage of lispro insulin is that it is very short acting and will not overlap with the next dose. Therefore some longer acting insulin needs to be given in order to provide the basal or background insulin needs between meals and during the night. This can be done by administering 2 injections a day of NPH or lente insulin or one or two injections a day of ultralente. The lispro is then given three times a day with each meal. The insulin has been thoroughly tested in worldwide studies and the data will shortly be submitted to the Food and Drug Administration for their approval. When approved by the FDA the insulin will then be available on the market as a new adjunct to treatment which should improve and enhance our ability to provide more efficient, flexible and smoother intensive insulin therapy in keeping with the mandates of the Diabetes Control and Complications Trial (DCCT).

The Question Regarding Non-Invasive Blood Glucose Monitoring

Noninvasive blood glucose monitoring is a technology whose time has come. The technology is simple and has been available for some time. It involves the passing into the body a beam of light that is close to the infrared spectrum. A laser generated infrared beam can be passed into a potato or an apple or some other object and this beam of light will set to vibrating the various molecules. Since the molecules vibrate at different frequencies, that is water, sugar, fat, amino acids, etc. are all vibrating, but vibrating at different frequencies, one can then attache a tuner or receiver and tune it to the frequency that you want. We can tune to the frequency of sugar and then the amplitude of that signal which comes back to the receiver will tell you how much of the sugar is present. This technology was developed originally for the food industry to determine the sugar content of potatoes and of orchard fruit prior to picking. It has now been adapted by a number of companies who are working on models to measure the sugar in blood by passing the beam through the skin.

Initial models attempting to use the finger have not been successful as yet because of the variation of the thickness of skin which can vary due to frequent past blood glucose testing and from occupational hazards which can increase the thickness of the skin. Diasense, Inc. of Pittsburg, PA, has developed a model called Diasense 1000 which was submitted to the FDA for approval in January, 1994 and should be available on the market in the near future. This model measures the blood sugar through the skin in the soft underpart of the forearm. Since everybody's skin is approximately the same thickness there, there is not as much problem with standardization. The disadvantage of this machine, which is highly accurate, is that it is stationary. It is not portable. It is a 110 volt AC machine which has to be plugged in. It is the size of a bread box and is fairly heavy. Therefore, it is a home model not a portable unit which can be carried with you to test the blood sugar. It has on it a rounded, cup-shaped area that the arm will fit into. The beam of light is then passed in and the blood sugar is then read. The initial model will be fairly expensive with the price approaching $8,000. There are a number of companies working on other models, including direct current models, which are smaller and more portable. As more companies come out with their units the price of all units should begin to decline. This is, however, the technology of the future and should be looked for with hope.

Update for Management of Type I Diabetes

The attitude toward the management of type I diabetes and to a lesser extent type II diabetes has been greatly changed by the Diabetes Control and Complications Trial (DCCT) which has shown conclusively that we need to obtain and maintain a high degree of control in order to prevent complications of diabetes. This has resulted in a great impetus to develop new methods of management. Various people are searching for new ways to provide this management using various kinds of protocols, algorithms and mathematical formulas. It has been shown that the exchange system does not fit well into this kind of management, so new dietary regimens or methodologies are being searched for and researched in order to improve control.

However, the techniques for really good control in keeping with the DCCT focus and principles have really been discussed in the past. They are 1) the care of the individual with diabetes by an especially trained team, that is educated and experienced in the management of type I diabetes; 2) education of the patient in all aspects of diabetes including principles of self management so that the patient can become empowered to take responsibility for their own care; 3) the use of a flexible dietary program which will match the insulin administration and, finally; 4) a flexible multi-dose insulin regimen which then can be modified to fit the various lifestyles and changing lifestyles of individuals with diabetes. These are the principles which have and will guide the development of methodologies for managing type I diabetes.

As far as type II diabetes is concerned, the evidence indicates that the people also need to be kept under better control and this will lead to changing more individuals to insulin earlier and the use of multiple dose insulin regimes more frequently in Type II diabetes. A new drug which will soon be available is Metformin or Glucophage. Metformin is not a new drug. It has been used in most of the rest of the world for the last 30 years. It is new to the United States however, and will be on the market soon. It is currently available through an investigational new drug number which any experienced dietologist can obtain through application but it will be available for commercial use in a few months. This drug works differently than the other oral hypoglycemic agents therefore it can be used either alone or in conjunction with the present drugs. It should enhance therapy, providing not only better control, but a longer time period of being able to use oral hyperglycemic agents before a change to insulin.

All this, however, has led to the need for more self blood glucose monitoring in people with Type II diabetes so that these various medications can be individualized to meet the specific needs of individuals and to meet their needs as those needs change. Without self blood glucose monitoring medication cannot be tailored to the needs of the individual and the kind of control necessary to meet the standards of the DCCT cannot be obtained. Therefore, it is our feeling that all diabetic patients should be well educated and should be doing self blood glucose monitoring.

Funding for Research

Besides the National Institutes of Health, the major funders of diabetes research are the American Diabetes Association and the Juvenile Diabetes Foundation. Still, the funds are not enough to support the many new ideas that are submitted for funding purposes. Funds are needed for salaries, for equipment, for supplies, and for the paperwork involved in reporting and sharing the information from investigator to investigator and from the research centers to the public. Training funds are needed to develop the researchers of tomorrow. By the time a physician or other scientist completes the necessary research preparation, most of the funds have been used up.

For the physician, an offer of a medical practice often takes the place of research work so that he or she can have enough of an income.

Research training programs need supplies and equipment. Sometimes this equipment needs to be constructed to meet the researchers' guidelines (for example, in the case of the implantable artificial pancreas, no equipment was available to proceed with such an idea, so the machine had to be made from the ground up).

To aid research efforts, talk with your legislators and encourage an increase in funding for diabetes research. Support your diabetes association and their fund-raising efforts, and aid them in their efforts to alert the public to the dangers of diabetes and the need for research support.

The need for research into diabetes will be with us until the disease has finally been conquered. At present, education and knowledge are our best weapons. The more you, as an individual, keep yourself fit by following your program, the better able you will be to benefit from new research. And the more you share your ideas on the prevention, cure, or treatment of the disease with health professionals or the diabetes association, the more you will be helping to make diabetes mellitus become a disease of the past.

Appendix A

Food Questionnaire

Phone: _____ Physician: _____

Name: _____ Birthdate: _____

Address: _____ Spouse: _____

How much milk do you drink a day? _____

Do you use butter? _____ or margarine? _____

If you use bread, what kind? White _____ Whole grain _____

If you use tortillas, what kind? Flour _____ Corn _____

If you use rice, what kind? White _____ Brown _____

Do you use kosher foods? Always _____ Sometimes _____ Never _____

How many times a week do you eat the following foods:

Name of food	Never	4 or more times a week?	Daily?	How much is a serving?
Hard cheese	_____	_____	_____	_____ Slices
Eggs	_____	_____	_____	_____ Whole
Steak, hamburger, pork chops, etc.	_____	_____	_____	_____ Ounces
Cold cuts, hot dogs, sausage, or luncheon meats	_____	_____	_____	_____ Pieces/ Ounces
Pizza	_____	_____	_____	_____ Pieces
Sweet rolls, doughnuts	_____	_____	_____	_____ Pieces
Deep-fat fried foods (french fries, etc.)	_____	_____	_____	_____ Pieces
Soda pop (diet or not)	_____	_____	_____	_____ Cups

Fruit drink (NOT fruit juice)	____	____	____	____	Cups
Alcoholic beverages (beer, wine, whiskey, cocktails, etc.)	____	____	____	____	Cups/oz
Milk shakes, ice cream, etc.	____	____	____	____	Cups
Candy	____	____	____	____	Pieces
Potato chips, other chips	____	____	____	____	Whole pieces
Crackers, pretzels	____	____	____	____	Whole pieces
Hot breads	____	____	____	____	Whole pieces
Vegetables (dark green or deep yellow)	____	____	____	____	Cups
Citrus fruits (orange, grapefruit, tangerine, or tomato)	____	____	____	____	Cups
Potato	____	____	____	____	Whole
Sweet potato, yam	____	____	____	____	Whole
Corn, hominy	____	____	____	____	Cups
Other fruits and vegetables	____	____	____	____	Cups
Fish (including tuna)	____	____	____	____	Ounces
Chicken, turkey, other fowl	____	____	____	____	Ounces
Lean meat	____	____	____	____	Ounces
Cottage cheese or yogurt	____	____	____	____	Cups
Macaroni, noodles, spaghetti	____	____	____	____	Cups
Cereal, cooked	____	____	____	____	Cups
Cereal, dry	____	____	____	____	Cups
Corn bread, biscuits, bagels, muffins, waffles, pancakes	____	____	____	____	Whole pieces

Breads, buns, tortillas	___	___	___	___ Slices
Jelly, honey, jam, syrup, preserves	___	___	___	___ Tbsp
Tofu, nuts/seeds	___	___	___	___ Tbsp
Bacon, salt pork	___	___	___	___ Slices
Peanut butter	___	___	___	___ Tbsp
Baked or cooked beans (pinto, navy, butter, lima, split peas, lentil)	___	___	___	___ Cups
Soybeans	___	___	___	___ Cups
Salad dressing, mayonnaise	___	___	___	___ Tbsp
Rice, grits	___	___	___	___ Cups
Popcorn	___	___	___	___ Cups
Catsup	___	___	___	___ Tbsp
Molasses, sorghum	___	___	___	___ Tbsp
Chili	___	___	___	___ Cups
Sweetened gelatin or Popsicles	___	___	___	___ Cups
Pudding, custards, condensed milk	___	___	___	___ Cups
Cream	___	___	___	___ Tbsp
Gravy	___	___	___	___ Tbsp
Soup	___	___	___	___ Cups
Soup with milk	___	___	___	___ Cups
Olives, pickles	___	___	___	___ Pieces
Coffee, tea	___	___	___	___ Cups
Cocoa, chocolate	___	___	___	___ Cups
Chinese foods (chow mein, chop suey, etc.)	___	___	___	___ Cups
Italian foods (lasagna, spaghetti with meat balls, etc.)	___	___	___	___ Cups
Taco, enchiladas, tamales, etc.	___	___	___	___ Whole pieces
Macaroni and cheese	___	___	___	___ Cups

List other foods NOT listed above that you regularly eat:

_____

_____

_____

Circle what you use for seasoning foods:
Salt in cooking, salt at table, monosodium glutamate, meat tenderizer, soy sauce,

Tabasco, other: _____

Circle the foods you like:
apricots, artichokes, avocados, bananas, bean sprouts, beets, bok choy, broccoli,
brussels sprouts, cabbage, cantaloupe, carrots, green peppers, greens, mangoes,
papayas, peas, raisins, radishes, sauerkraut, scallions, spinach, strawberries,

Swiss chard, turnips, watermelon, squash (kind) _____

Appendix B

FOOD AND NUTRITION BOARD, NATIONAL ACADEMY OF SCIENCES—NATIONAL RESEARCH COUNCIL
RECOMMENDED DIETARY ALLOWANCES,[a] Revised 1989

Designed for the maintenance of good nutrition of practically all healthy people in the United States

Category	Age (years) or Condition	Weight[b] (kg)	(lb)	Height[b] (cm)	(in)	Protein (g)	Fat-Soluble Vitamins			
							Vitamin A (µg RE)[c]	Vitamin D (µg)[d]	Vitamin E (mg α-TE)[e]	Vitamin K (µg)
Infants	0.0–0.5	6	13	60	24	13	375	7.5	3	5
	0.5–1.0	9	20	71	28	14	375	10	4	10
Children	1–3	13	29	90	35	16	400	10	6	15
	4–6	20	44	112	44	24	500	10	7	20
	7–10	28	62	132	52	28	700	10	7	30
Males	11–14	45	99	157	62	45	1,000	10	10	45
	15–18	66	145	176	69	59	1,000	10	10	65
	19–24	72	160	177	70	58	1,000	10	10	70
	25–50	79	174	176	70	63	1,000	5	10	80
	51+	77	170	173	68	63	1,000	5	10	80
Females	11–14	46	101	157	62	46	800	10	8	45
	15–18	55	120	163	64	44	800	10	8	55
	19–24	58	128	164	65	46	800	10	8	60
	25–50	63	138	163	64	50	800	5	8	65
	51+	65	143	160	63	50	800	5	8	65
Pregnant						60	800	10	10	65
Lactating	1st 6 months					65	1,300	10	12	65
	2nd 6 months					62	1,200	10	11	65

RECOMMENDED DIETARY ALLOWANCES (continued)

Water-Soluble Vitamins

Category	Age (years) or Condition	Weight (kg)	(lb)	Height (cm)	(in)	Vitamin C (mg)	Thiamin (mg)	Riboflavin (mg)	Niacin (mg NE)	Vitamin B$_6$ (mg)	Folate (µg)	Vitamin B$_{12}$ (µg)
Infants	0.0–0.5	6	13	60	24	30	0.3	0.4	5	0.3	25	0.3
	0.5–1.0	9	20	71	28	35	0.4	0.5	6	0.6	35	0.5
Children	1–3	13	29	90	35	40	0.7	0.8	9	1.0	50	0.7
	4–6	20	44	112	44	45	0.9	1.1	12	1.1	75	1.0
	7–10	28	62	132	52	45	1.0	1.2	13	1.4	100	1.4
Males	11–14	45	99	157	62	50	1.3	1.5	17	1.7	150	2.0
	15–18	66	145	176	69	60	1.5	1.8	20	2.0	200	2.0
	19–24	72	160	177	70	60	1.5	1.7	19	2.0	200	2.0
	25–50	79	174	176	70	60	1.5	1.7	19	2.0	200	2.0
	51+	77	170	173	68	60	1.2	1.4	15	2.0	200	2.0
Females	11–14	46	101	157	62	50	1.1	1.3	15	1.4	150	2.0
	15–18	55	120	163	64	60	1.1	1.3	15	1.5	180	2.0
	19–24	58	128	164	65	60	1.1	1.3	15	1.6	180	2.0
	25–50	63	138	163	64	60	1.1	1.3	15	1.6	180	2.0
	51+	65	143	160	63	60	1.0	1.2	13	1.6	180	2.0
Pregnant						70	1.5	1.6	17	2.2	400	2.2
Lactating	1st 6 months					95	1.6	1.8	20	2.1	280	2.6
	2nd 6 months					90	1.6	1.7	20	2.1	260	2.6

RECOMMENDED DIETARY ALLOWANCES *(continued)*

Minerals

Category	Age (years) or Condition	Weight[b] (kg)	Weight[b] (lb)	Height[b] (cm)	Height[b] (in)	Calcium (mg)	Phosphorus (mg)	Magnesium (mg)	Iron (mg)	Zinc (mg)	Iodine (µg)	Selenium (µg)
Infants	0.0–0.5	6	13	60	24	400	300	40	6	5	40	10
	0.5–1.0	9	20	71	28	600	500	60	10	5	50	15
Children	1–3	13	29	90	35	800	800	80	10	10	70	20
	4–6	20	44	112	44	800	800	120	10	10	90	20
	7–10	28	62	132	52	800	800	170	10	10	120	30
Males	11–14	45	99	157	62	1,200	1,200	270	12	15	150	40
	15–18	66	145	176	69	1,200	1,200	400	12	15	150	50
	19–24	72	160	177	70	1,200	1,200	350	10	15	150	70
	25–50	79	174	176	70	800	800	350	10	15	150	70
	51+	77	170	173	68	800	800	350	10	15	150	70
Females	11–14	46	101	157	62	1,200	1,200	280	15	12	150	45
	15–18	55	120	163	64	1,200	1,200	300	15	12	150	50
	19–24	58	128	164	65	1,200	1,200	280	15	12	150	55
	25–50	63	138	163	64	800	800	280	15	12	150	55
	51+	65	143	160	63	800	800	280	10	12	150	55
Pregnant						1,200	1,200	320	30	15	175	65
Lactating	1st 6 months					1,200	1,200	355	15	19	200	75
	2nd 6 months					1,200	1,200	340	15	16	200	75

aThe allowances, expressed as average daily intakes over time, are intended to provide for individual variations among most normal persons as they live in the United States under usual environmental stresses. Diets should be based on a variety of common foods in order to provide other nutrients for which human requirements have been less well defined.

bWeights and heights of Reference Adults are actual medians for the U.S. population of the designated age, as reported by NHANES II. The median weights and heights of those under 19 years of age were taken from Hamill et al. (1979) (see pages 16–17). The use of these figures does not imply that the height-to-weight ratios are ideal.

cRetinol equivalents. 1 retinol equivalent = 1 µg retinol or 6 µg β-carotene.

dAs cholecalciferol. 10 µg cholecalciferol = 400 IU of vitamin D.

eα-Tocopherol equivalents. 1 mg d-α tocopherol = 1 α-TE.

f1 NE (niacin equivalent) is equal to 1 mg of niacin or 60 mg of dietary tryptophan.

RECOMMENDED DIETARY ALLOWANCES (CONTINUED)
SUMMARY TABLE
Estimated Safe and Adequate Daily Dietary Intakes of Selected Vitamins and Minerals[a]

Category	Age (years)	Vitamins		Trace Elements[b]				
		Biotin (µg)	Pantothenic Acid (mg)	Copper (mg)	Manganese (mg)	Fluoride (mg)	Chromium (µg)	Molybdenum (µg)
Infants	0–0.5	10	2	0.4–0.6	0.3–0.6	0.1–0.5	10–40	15–30
	0.5–1	15	3	0.6–0.7	0.6–1.0	0.2–1.0	20–60	20–40
Children and adolescents	1–3	20	3	0.7–1.0	1.0–1.5	0.5–1.5	20–80	25–50
	4–6	25	3–4	1.0–1.5	1.5–2.0	1.0–2.5	30–120	30–75
	7–10	30	4–5	1.0–2.0	2.0–3.0	1.5–2.5	50–200	50–150
	11+	30–100	4–7	1.5–2.5	2.0–5.0	1.5–2.5	50–200	75–250
Adults		30–100	4–7	1.5–3.0	2.0–5.0	1.5–4.0	50–200	75–250

[a]Because there is less information on which to base allowances, these figures are not given in the main table of RDA and are provided here in the form of ranges of recommended intakes.

[b]Since the toxic levels for many trace elements may be only several times usual intakes, the upper levels for the trace elements given in this table should not be habitually exceeded.

Appendix C

*American Diabetes Association Exchange Lists**

The following Exchange Lists have been included but other recommendations may be forthcoming from the American Diabetes Association in cooperation with the American Dietetic Association. These associations are working on revising the dietary guidelines which should be available sometime during 1995. The emphasis will be on individual consultation with a registered dietitian. It also supports the concept that a meal plan must be tailored to the type of diabetes, the method of treatment and whether the person has a weight problem or not. Other dietary problems would also be addressed (i.e. cholesterol problems, etc.). Learning a baseline meal plan and following such a plan as much as possible is essential in successfully achieving normal blood glucose levels.

A total amount of carbohydrate in the diet rather than the source seems to be the factor that influences after meal blood sugar levels. If table sugar (sucrose) is used as part of the meal plan, blood glucose is not necessarily effected. If used alone or added to the meal, it will account for elevated blood sugar levels. This does not say the one can freely use table sugar. It is saying that sugar can be eaten in modest amounts but as part of a balanced meal plan.

---

*The Exchange Lists are the basis of a meal planning system designed by a committee of the American Diabetes Association and The American Dietetic Association. While designed primarily for people with diabetes and others who must follow special diets, the Exchange Lists are based on principles of good nutrition that apply to everyone. © 1986 American Diabetes Association, The American Dietetic Association.

There are a variety of approaches to meal planning. One newer one is called, "Carbohydrate Counting." This is helpful for many people, but for growing children and others, recognition of total caloric intake and content in the basic meal plan is a must. The Pyramid is also being used by many. This follows general recommendations as found in most meal plans: cereals, breads, rice, potatoes, and pasta form the base of the pyramid. The second level includes fruits and vegetables; the third dairy products, meat, fish, and eggs. The top part includes fats and sweets with the admonition to use sparingly (i.e. less than 30% of the diet should be used as Fat).

Weight loss is supported but the focus on ideal body weight to height is not the goal as much as such was before. It has been found that a mild to moderate weight loss of 10–20 pounds has been shown to improve diabetes control. The goal is now focused on a healthy body weight with the purpose to achieve desired blood sugar and lipid (fat or cholesterol and triglyceride) levels. You may obtain a copy of the new nutrition guidelines by contacting the Order Fulfillment Dept. at the American Diabetes Association's National Center at 1-800-232-3472.

When you have diabetes, your body can't use the food you eat in the proper way. When you eat, food is digested and much of it is changed into glucose, a sugar the body uses for fuel. The glucose is carried by the bloodstream to the individual cells of the body. The body produces a hormone called insulin that helps the glucose enter the cells. Normally, enough insulin is produced to allow the glucose in the blood to be absorbed by the cells, where it is used for energy. Insulin also helps the body to store extra glucose and fat for later use.

When you have diabetes, your body does not make enough, or any, insulin, or does not use it properly. Without insulin, your body cannot use the food you eat. The digested food, in the form of glucose, builds up in your blood. The cells can't get the energy they need, because insulin isn't available to move the glucose into the cells. The symptoms of diabetes are caused by the high blood-glucose levels. People with diabetes may also have high blood-fat levels (cholesterol and triglycerides). Over time, higher than normal blood-glucose and blood-fat levels may cause serious long-term complications.

There are two major types of diabetes mellitus:

insulin-dependent (IDDM, Type I, juvenile onset)

non–insulin-dependent (NIDDM, Type II, adult onset)

People with **insulin-dependent diabetes** do not make insulin. When the body has no insulin and cannot use glucose for energy, it begins to burn fat. When fat is burned for energy, acid wastes called ketones are formed. The ketones build up in the blood and cause a serious condition called ketoacidosis. People with insulin-dependent diabetes must take insulin injections to avoid this life-threatening condition.

People with **non–insulin-dependent diabetes** make some insulin, but there either is not enough or it does not work properly. This type of diabetes can often be controlled through diet and exercise. Oral hypoglycemic agents (diabetes pills) help some people to make more insulin or to use their own insulin better. Some people with non–insulin-dependent diabetes may need insulin injections to regulate their blood-glucose levels.

Managing Diabetes with Food

The management of diabetes has three parts: food, activity, and medication (if needed). Food raises blood-glucose and blood-fat levels. Activity and medications (insulin or oral hypoglycemic agents) lower blood-glucose and blood-fat levels. A balance of these three parts leads to good management of diabetes. In this section, our focus will be on food.

The nutritional goals of diabetes management are appropriate blood-glucose and blood-fat levels. You will learn to balance the food you eat with your activity level and with the insulin in your body so that the levels of glucose and fats (cholesterol and triglycerides) in your blood stay as close to normal as possible. It is important to keep blood-glucose levels near normal to prevent problems that can result from too high a level (ketoacidosis or diabetic coma) or, if insulin is used, from too low a level (insulin reactions). It is important to match the amount of food you eat with the amount of insulin in your body, whether your body produces insulin (on its own or with the help of diabetes pills) or your insulin comes from injections. This will not only help you feel better (the symptoms of diabetes should disappear), but more importantly, it may also help to reduce or prevent the complications of diabetes.

Blood-glucose monitoring can be very useful in keeping track of your diabetes and can show you the effects of certain foods or activities on your blood-glucose levels. You can measure your own blood glucose using a finger-stick device and test strip. Your monitoring record will help you match your meal plan to other aspects of your diabetes management.

It is also important to limit the amount of fat in your diet, because higher levels of blood fats are associated with heart disease. People with diabetes run a greater risk of developing heart disease than other people.

Maintaining a Reasonable Weight

It is important to eat the right amount of calories to help you reach and stay at a reasonable body weight. The number of calories you need depends on your size, age, and activity level.

Eating too many calories causes weight gain, which will worsen diabetes and increase your risks for high blood pressure and heart disease. Your body makes and/or uses insulin best when you are at your desirable weight.

Eating too few calories causes a different problem. Children and teens with diabetes must eat enough calories to grow properly. Pregnant and nursing women must eat enough calories to provide for proper development of their babies.

Exercise is very important, too. It is helpful in weight loss, and it is also good for your heart and blood vessels. You can increase your activity level by walking, biking, or just taking the stairs instead of an elevator. If you wish to begin an exercise training program, check with your health-care team first.

Following Principles of Good Nutrition

It is important to eat a variety of foods each day. Your body works better if you eat a balanced diet that includes the right amounts of vitamins, minerals, carbohydrate, protein, and fat. Carbohydrate is the major source of energy. Protein builds muscle and tissue and provides some energy. Fat is the storage form of energy. Most foods contain a mixture of these. Carbohydrate, which has four calories per gram of weight, is found in starches, bread, fruit, vegetables, and milk. Protein also has four calories per gram of weight. Protein is found in meat and milk, and small amounts of it are found in starches, bread, and vegetables. Fat is higher in calories, with nine calories per gram of weight. Fat is found in meat, dairy products, oils, and nuts. Insulin is needed to use carbohydrate, protein, and fat properly.

Some principles of good nutrition:

Eat less fat. The average American adult eats too much fat. Too much fat may cause heart and blood-vessel disease. Eat fish, poultry, and other lean meats. Watch your portion sizes with all meat—it's easy to eat too much. Eat fewer high-fat foods, such as cold cuts, bacon, nuts, gravy, salad dressing, margarine, and solid shortening. Drink skim or low-fat milk and eat less ice cream, butter, and cheese.

Eat more carbohydrates (starches and breads), especially those high in fiber. Carbohydrate foods are a good source of energy, vitamins, and minerals. Fiber in foods may help to lower blood-glucose and blood-fat levels. All people should increase the amount of carbohydrate and fiber they eat. This can be done by eating more dried beans, peas, and lentils; more whole-grain breads, cereals, and crackers; and more fruits and vegetables. (Foods that are high in fiber will be noted later on with a special symbol: ¶.)

Eat less sugar. All people, not just those with diabetes, should eat less sugar. Sugar has lots of calories and no vitamins or minerals, and it causes cavities. Foods high in sugar include desserts (for example, frosted cake and pie), sugary breakfast foods, table sugar, honey, and syrup. One 12-ounce can of a regular soft drink has nine teaspoons of sugar!

Use less salt. Most of us eat too much salt. The sodium in salt can cause the body to retain water, and in some people it may raise blood pressure. Try to use less salt in cooking and at the table. Foods that are high in sodium, such as processed and convenience foods, will be noted later with a special symbol: §.)

Use alcohol in moderation. It is best to avoid alcohol altogether, but if you like to have an alcoholic drink now and then, ask your dietitian how to work it into your meal plan. If you take insulin, it is important to eat food with your drink.

How can I accomplish these goals?

A diabetes meal plan and the exchange lists will help you to meet all these goals. The first step is to talk to your dietitian, who will determine your daily nutritional needs and help you work out your own nutritional prescription. This prescription will match the calories, carbohydrate, protein, and fat you eat with your own activity levels and with the insulin in your body.

What is a diabetes meal plan?

You and your dietitian will work out a specific meal plan for you. Your meal plan is a guide that shows the number of food choices (exchanges) you can eat at each meal and snack. Your meal plan is designed so that more than half of your total daily calories will be carbohydrate, with less fat and protein consumed.

What are exchange lists?

Foods that are alike are grouped together in lists. The six exchange lists help to make your meal plan work. All the foods on a list have about the same amount of carbohydrate, protein, fat, and calories. In the amounts given, all the choices on each list are equal. Any food on a list can be exchanged or traded for any other food on the same list.

The six lists are: starch/bread, meat and substitutes, vegetables, fruit, milk, and fat.

The exchange lists and the meal plan will provide you with a great variety of food choices, and they will help you to control the distribution of calories, carbohydrate, protein, and fat throughout the day so that your food and your insulin will be balanced. This balance is what gives you good blood-glucose control.

Are meal plans different for different types of diabetes?

Yes, they are. The goals of treatment are somewhat different for the two types of diabetes.

INSULIN-DEPENDENT DIABETES.   The most important nutrition principle for people with insulin-dependent diabetes is *consistency*. Meals should be eaten at about the same time each day. The amounts and types of food eaten at each meal should be about the same from day to day. This is important, because the food you eat is planned to balance your insulin injections and your activity. Your meal plan and the exchange lists can help work together to regulate your blood-glucose levels. If your meal plan and your insulin are out of balance, wide swings in blood-glucose levels can occur, and you may suffer from insulin reactions or from the symptoms of high blood-glucose levels.

NON–INSULIN-DEPENDENT DIABETES.   Most people with non–insulin-dependent diabetes are overweight. Thus, the most important nutrition principle for people with this type of diabetes is weight control. You can lose weight by eating less food and increasing your exercise. It is still important to eat a balanced diet, even while losing weight. Your dietitian will help you to determine the number of calories you need and set weight goals, and will give you tips to help you reach these goals.

Do I have to change the way I now eat?

You may have to change the way you eat. Many people ask if they can eat the same foods as the rest of their family. The diabetes meal plan is not much different from the way everyone *should* eat. However, it is true that many people do not eat in such a healthful way. And it's very hard to change habits, especially about food. Just remember: make changes gradually, set short-term goals, and reward yourself when you are successful.

To make your meal plan work, you will need to eat what is prescribed for you. Serving sizes are very important to the success of your meal plan. If you eat too much food or too little food, your blood-glucose regulation and your weight will be affected. To help you estimate serving sizes accurately, you will need to measure or weigh your food for the first week or so, and again periodically as time goes on to see how you're doing. Suggestions for how to measure your serving sizes are included in the "Management Tips" section.

It is very important to see your dietitian regularly when you are first learning how to use your meal plan and exchange lists. Your meal plan can be adjusted if it is not working for you. The only way to make it right is to see your dietitian and solve the problems.

Will this meal plan always be right for me?

Your meal plan may need to be changed as time goes on. Changes in lifestyle (for example, those involving work, school, vacation, or travel) require adjustments in your meal plan. Your weight may change, your eating habits may change, or your activity may change—and any of these changes means you may need a new meal plan. As children grow they need more calories, and when they reach adulthood they need fewer. Check in with your dietitian regularly to review your meal plan, ask any questions you may have, and learn about new nutrition information. Regular nutrition counseling can help you make positive changes in your eating habits.

Remember, your meal plan is written just for you. It is intended to help you achieve your nutrition goals, and it takes your likes and dislikes into account. It is flexible and can be adjusted for your varying needs. You *can* change your eating habits. You'll feel better and be healthier, too. Good luck, and good eating!

The Exchange Lists

The reason for dividing food into six different groups is that foods vary in their carbohydrate, protein, fat, and calorie content. Each exchange list contains foods that are alike; each food choice on a list contains about the same amount of carbohydrate, protein, fat, and calories as the other choices on that list.

The following chart shows the amounts of nutrients in one serving from each exchange list. As you read the exchange lists, you will notice that one choice is often a larger amount of food than another choice from the same list. Because foods are so different, each food is measured or weighed so the amounts of carbohydrate, protein, fat, and calories are the same in each choice.

	Carbohydrate (grams)	Protein (grams)	Fat (grams)	Calories
I. Starch/Bread	15	3	trace	80
II. Meat				
Lean	—	7	3	55
Medium-Fat	—	7	5	75
High-Fat	—	7	8	100
III. Vegetable	5	2	—	25
IV. Fruit	15	—	—	60
V. Milk				
Skim	12	8	trace	90
Low-fat	12	8	5	120
Whole	12	8	8	120
VI. Fat	—	—	5	45

You will notice symbols on some foods in the exchange groups. Foods that are high in fiber (three grams or more per normal serving) have the symbol ¶. High-fiber foods are good for you, and it is important to eat more of these foods.

Foods that are high in sodium (400 milligrams or more of sodium per normal serving) have the symbol §. As noted, it's a good idea to limit your intake of high-salt foods, especially if you have high blood pressure.

If you have a favorite food that is not included in any of these groups, ask your dietitian about it. That food can probably be worked into your meal plan, at least now and then.

I. Starch/Bread List

Each item in this list contains approximately fifteen grams of carbohydrate, three grams of protein, a trace of fat, and eighty calories. Whole-grain products average about two grams of fiber per serving. Some foods are higher in fiber. Those foods that contain three or more grams of fiber per serving are identified with the symbol ¶.

You can choose your starch exchanges from any of the items on this list. If you want to eat a starch food that is not on the list, the general rule is this:

½ cup of cereal, grain, or pasta = one serving

1 ounce of a bread product = one serving

Your dietitian can help you to be more exact.

CEREALS/GRAINS/PASTA

¶ Bran cereals, concentrated (such as Bran Buds, All Bran)	⅓ cup
¶ Bran cereals, flaked	½ cup
Bulgur (cooked)	½ cup
Cooked cereals	½ cup
Cornmeal (dry)	2½ tbsp
Grape Nuts	3 tbsp
Grits (cooked)	½ cup
Other ready-to-eat, unsweetened cereals	¾ cup
Pasta (cooked)	½ cup
Puffed cereal	1½ cups
Rice, white or brown (cooked)	⅓ cup
Shredded wheat	½ cup
¶ Wheat germ	3 tbsp

DRIED BEANS/PEAS/LENTILS

¶ Beans and peas (cooked) (such as kidney, white, split, blackeye)	⅓ cup
¶ Lentils (cooked)	⅓ cup
¶ Baked beans	¼ cup

STARCHY VEGETABLES

(¶ = 3 grams or more of fiber per serving)

¶ Corn	½ cup
¶ Corn on the cob, 6 in. long	1
¶ Lima beans	½ cup
¶ Peas, green (canned or frozen)	½ cup
¶ Plaintain	½ cup
Potato, baked	1 small (3 oz)
Potato, mashed	½ cup
Squash, winter (acorn, butternut)	¾ cup
Yam, sweet potato (plain)	⅓ cup

BREAD

Bagel	½ (1 oz)
Bread sticks, crisp, 4 in. long x ½ in.	2 (⅔ oz)
Croutons, low fat	1 cup
English muffin	½
Frankfurter or hamburger bun	½ (1 oz)
Pita, 6 in. across	½
Plain roll, small	1 (1 oz)

Raisin, unfrosted	1 slice	
¶ Rye, pumpernickel	1 slice (1 oz)	
Tortilla, 6 in. across	1	
White (including French, Italian)	1 slice (1 oz)	
Whole wheat	1 slice	

CRACKERS/SNACKS

Animal crackers	8
Graham crackers, 2½ in. square	3
Matzoh	¾ oz
Melba toast	5 slices
Oyster crackers	24
Popcorn (popped, no fat added)	3 cups
Pretzels	¾ oz
Rye crisp (2 in. x 3½ in.)	4
Saltine-type crackers	6
Whole-wheat crackers, no fat added (crisp breads such as Finn, Kavli, Wasa)	2–4 slices (¾ oz)

STARCHY FOODS PREPARED WITH FAT (count as 1 starch/bread serving, plus 1 fat serving)

Biscuit, 2½ in. across	1
Chow mein noodles	½ cup
Corn bread, 2-in. cube	1 (2 oz)
Cracker, round butter type	6
French-fried potatoes (2 in. to 3½ in. long)	10 (1½ oz)
Muffin, plain, small	1
Pancake, 4 in. across	2
Stuffing, bread (prepared)	¼ cup
Taco shell, 6 in. across	2
Waffle, 4½ in. square	1
Whole-wheat crackers, fat added (such as Triscuits)	4–6 (1 oz)

II. Meat List

Each serving of meat and substitutes on this list contains about seven grams of protein. The amount of fat and number of calories vary, depending on what kind of meat or substitute is chosen. The list is divided into three parts, based on the amount of fat and calories: lean meat, medium-fat meat, and high-fat meat. One ounce (one meat exchange) of each of these includes the following nutrient amounts:

	Carbohydrate (grams)	Protein (grams)	Fat (grams)	Calories
Lean	0	7	3	55
Medium-fat	0	7	5	75
High-fat	0	7	8	100

You are encouraged to use more lean and medium-fat meat, poultry, and fish in your meal plan. This will help you to decrease your fat intake, which may help decrease your risk for heart disease. The items from the high-fat group are high in saturated fat, cholesterol, and calories. You should limit your choices from the high-fat group to three times per week. Meat and substitutes do not contribute any fiber to your meal plan. Meats and meat substitutes that have 400 milligrams or more of sodium per exchange are indicated with the symbol §.

Tips

1. Bake, roast, broil, grill, or boil these foods rather than frying them with added fat.

2. Use a nonstick pan spray or a nonstick pan to brown or fry these foods.

3. Trim off visible fat before and after cooking.

4. Do not add flour, bread crumbs, coating mixes, or fat to these foods when preparing them.

5. Weigh meat after removing bones and fat and again after cooking. Three ounces of cooked meat are equal to about four ounces of raw meat. Some examples of meat portions are:
   2 ounces meat (2 meat exchanges) = 1 small chicken leg or thigh, ½ cup cottage cheese or tuna
   3 ounces meat (3 meat exchanges) = 1 medium pork chop, 1 small hamburger, ½ of a whole chicken breast, 1 unbreaded fish fillet, cooked meat, about the size of a deck of cards

6. Restaurants usually serve prime cuts of meat, which are high in fat and calories.

LEAN MEAT AND SUBSTITUTES
One exchange is equal to any one of the following items:

Beef	USDA Good or Choice grades of lean beef, such as round, sirloin, and flank steak; tenderloin; and chipped beef §	1 oz

Pork	Lean pork, such as fresh ham; canned, cured, or boiled ham §, Canadian bacon §, tenderloin	1 oz
Veal	All cuts are lean except for veal cutlets (ground or cubed)	1 oz
Poultry	Chicken, turkey, Cornish hen (without skin)	1 oz
Fish	All fresh and frozen fish	1 oz
	Crab, lobster, scallops, shrimp, clams (fresh or canned in water §)	2 oz
	Oysters	6 medium
	Tuna § (canned in water)	¼ cup
	Herring (uncreamed or smoked)	1 oz
	Sardines (canned)	2 medium
Wild Game	Venison, rabbit, squirrel	1 oz
	Pheasant, duck, goose (without skin)	1 oz
Cheese	Any cottage cheese	¼ cup
	Grated parmesan	2 tbsp
	Diet cheese § (with fewer than 55 calories per ounce)	1 oz
Other	95% fat-free luncheon meat	1 oz
	Egg whites	3
	Egg substitutes (with fewer than 55 calories per ¼ cup)	¼ cup

MEDIUM-FAT AND MEAT SUBSTITUTES
One exchange is equal to any one of the following items:

Beef	Most beef products fall into this category. Examples are: all ground beef, roast (rib, chuck, rump), steak (cubed, Porterhouse, T-bone), and meat loaf.	1 oz
Pork	Most pork products fall into this category (examples: chops, loin roast, Boston butt, cutlets)	1 oz
Lamb	Most lamb products fall into this category (examples: chops, leg, roast)	1 oz
Veal	Cutlet (ground or cubed, unbreaded)	1 oz
Poultry	Chicken (with skin), domestic duck or goose (well drained of fat), ground turkey	1 oz

Fish	Tuna § (canned in oil and drained)	¼ cup
	Salmon § (canned)	¼ cup
Cheese	Skim or part-skim milk cheeses, such as:	
	Ricotta	¼ cup
	Mozzarella	1 oz
	Diet cheeses § (with 56–80 calories per ounce)	1 oz
Other	86% fat-free luncheon meat §	1 oz
	Egg (high in cholesterol, so limit to 3 per week)	1
	Egg substitutes (with 56–80 calories per ¼ cup)	¼ cup
	Tofu (2½ in. x 2¾ in. x 1 in.)	4 oz
	Liver, heart, kidney, sweetbreads (high in cholesterol)	1 oz

HIGH-FAT MEAT AND SUBSTITUTES
**Remember, these items are high in saturated fat, cholesterol, and calories, and should be eaten only three times per week.
One exchange is equal to any one of the following items:**

Beef	Most USDA Prime cuts of beef, such as ribs, corned beef §	1 oz
Pork	Spareribs, ground pork, pork sausage § (patty or link)	1 oz
Lamb	Patties (ground lamb)	1 oz
Fish	Any fried fish product	1 oz
Cheese	All regular cheese §, such as American, Blue, Cheddar, Monterey, Swiss	1 oz
Other	Luncheon meat §, such as bologna, salami, pimiento loaf	1 oz
	Sausage §, such as Polish, Italian	1 oz
	Knockwurst, smoked	1 oz
	Bratwurst §	1 oz
	Frankfurter § (turkey or chicken) (10/lb)	1 frank
	Peanut butter (contains unsaturated fat)	1 tbsp

COUNT AS ONE HIGH-FAT MEAT PLUS ONE FAT EXCHANGE:

Frankfurter § (beef, pork, or combination) (10/lb.)	1 frank
§ (400 mg or more of sodium per exchange)	

III. Vegetable List

Each vegetable serving on this list contains about five grams of carbohydrate, two grams of protein, and twenty-five calories. Vegetables contain two to three grams of dietary fiber. Vegetables that contain 400 mg of sodium per serving are identified with a § symbol.

Vegetables are a good source of vitamins and minerals. Fresh and frozen vegetables have more vitamins and less added salt. Rinsing canned vegetables will remove much of the salt.

Unless otherwise noted, the serving size for vegetables (one vegetable exchange) is:

½ cup of cooked vegetables or vegetable juice

1 cup of raw vegetables

Artichoke (½ medium)	Mushrooms, cooked
Asparagus	Okra
Beans (green, wax, Italian)	Onions
Bean sprouts	Pea pods
Beets	Peppers (green)
Broccoli	Rutabaga
Brussels sprouts	Sauerkraut §
Cabbage, cooked	Spinach, cooked
Carrots	Summer squash (crookneck)
Cauliflower	Tomato (one large)
Eggplant	Tomato/vegetable juice §
Greens (collard, mustard, turnip)	Turnips
	Water chestnuts
Kohlrabi	Zucchini, cooked
Leeks	

Starchy vegetables such as corn, peas, and potatoes are found on the Starch/Bread List.

For "free" vegetables (i.e., fewer than ten calories per serving), see the Free Food List.

§ 400 mg or more of sodium per serving.

IV. Fruit List

Each item on this list contains about fifteen grams of carbohydrate and sixty calories. Fresh, frozen, and dry fruits have about two grams of fiber per serving. Fruits that have three or more grams of fiber per serving have a ¶ symbol. Fruit juices contain very little dietary fiber.

The carbohydrate and calorie contents for a fruit serving are based on the usual serving of the most commonly eaten fruits. Use fresh fruits or frozen or canned fruits with no sugar added. Whole fruit is more filling than fruit juice and may be a better choice for those who are trying to lose weight. Unless otherwise noted, the serving size for one fruit serving is:

½ cup of fresh fruit or fruit juice

¼ cup of dried fruit

FRESH, FROZEN, AND UNSWEETENED CANNED FRUIT

Apples (raw, 2 in. across)	1	Honeydew melon (medium)	⅛
Applesauce (unsweetened)	½ cup	(cubes)	1 cup
		Kiwi (large)	1 kiwi
Apricots (canned) (4 halves)	½ cup	Mandarin oranges	¾ cup
		Mango (small)	½
Banana (9 in. long)	½	Nectarines (2½ in. across)	1
Blackberries (raw)	¾ cup	Orange (2½ in. across)	1
¶ Blueberries (raw)	¾ cup		
Cantaloupe (5 in. across)	⅓	Papaya	1 cup
		Peach (2¾ in. across)	1 (¾ cup)
(cubes)	1 cup		
Cherries (large, raw)	12 whole	Peaches (canned) (2 halves)	1 cup
Cherries (canned)	½ cup	Pear (½ large)	1 small
Figs (raw, 2 in. across)	2	Pears (canned) (2 halves)	½ cup
Fruit cocktail (canned)	½ cup	Persimmon (medium, native)	2
Grapefruit (medium)	½	Pineapple (raw)	¾ cup
		Pineapple (canned)	⅓ cup
Grapefruit (segments)	¾ cup	Plum (raw, 2 in. across)	2
Grapes (small)	15	¶ Pomegranate	½

¶ Raspberries (raw)	1 cup	Raisins	2 tbsp
¶ Strawberries (raw, whole)	1¼ cups	**FRUIT JUICE**	
Tangerine (2½ in. across)	2	Apple juice/cider	½ cup
		Cranberry juice cocktail	⅓ cup
Watermelon (cubes)	1¼ cups		
		Grapefruit juice	½ cup
		Grape juice	⅓ cup
DRIED FRUIT ¶		Orange juice	½ cup
¶ Apples	4 rings	Pineapple juice	½ cup
¶ Apricots	7 halves	Prune juice	⅓ cup
Dates (medium)	2½	¶ 3 or more grams of fiber per serving	
¶ Figs	1½		
¶ Prunes (medium)	3		

V. Milk List

Each serving of milk or milk products on this list contains about twelve grams of carbohydrate and eight grams of protein. The amount of fat in milk is measured in percent of butterfat. The calories vary depending on the kind of milk chosen. The list is divided into three parts, based on the amount of fat and calories: skim/very low-fat milk, low-fat milk, and whole milk. One serving (one milk exchange) of each of these includes:

	Carbohydrate (grams)	Protein (grams)	Fat (grams)	Calories
Milk				
Skim	12	8	trace	90
Low-fat	12	8	5	140
Whole	12	8	8	160

Milk is the body's main source of calcium, the mineral needed for growth and repair of bones. Yogurt is also a good source of calcium. Yogurt and many dry or powdered milk products have different amounts of fat. If you have questions about a particular item, read the label to find out the fat and calorie content.

Milk can be drunk or added to cereal or other foods. Many tasty dishes, such as sugar-free pudding, are made with milk (see the Combination Foods list). Add life to plain yogurt by adding one of your fruit servings to it.

SKIM AND VERY LOW-FAT MILK

Skim milk	1 cup
½% milk	1 cup
1% milk	1 cup
Low-fat buttermilk	1 cup
Evaporated skim milk	½ cup
Dry nonfat milk	⅓ cup
Plain nonfat yogurt	8 oz

LOW-FAT MILK

2% milk	1 cup
Plain low-fat yogurt (with added nonfat milk solids)	8 oz

WHOLE MILK

The whole-milk group has much more fat per serving than the skim and low-fat groups. Whole milk has more than 3¼% butterfat. Try to limit your choices from the whole-milk group as much as possible.

Whole milk	1 cup
Evaporated whole milk	½ cup
Whole-milk plain yogurt	8 oz

VI. Fat List

Each serving on the fat list contains about five grams of fat and forty-five calories.

The foods on the fat list contain mostly fat, although some items may also contain a small amount of protein. All fats are high in calories and should be carefully measured. Everyone should modify fat intake by eating unsaturated fats instead of saturated fats. The sodium content of these foods varies widely. Check the label for sodium information.

UNSATURATED FATS

Avocado	⅛ medium	Peanuts (small)	20
Margarine	1 tsp	(large)	10
*Margarine, diet	1 tbsp	Walnuts	2 whole
Mayonnaise	1 tsp	Other nuts	1 tbsp
*Mayonnaise (reduced-calorie)	1 tbsp	Seeds (except pumpkin), pine nuts, sunflower	
Nuts and Seeds:		(without shells)	1 tbsp
Almonds, dry roasted	6	Pumpkin seeds	2 tsp
Cashews, dry roasted	1 tbsp	Oil (corn, cottonseed, safflower, soybean, sunflower, olive, peanut)	1 tsp
Pecans	2		

*Olives (small)	10	Chitterlings	½ oz
(large)	5	Coconut, shredded	2 tbsp
Salad dressing, mayonnaise-type, regular	2 tsp	Coffee whitener, liquid	2 tbsp
Salad dressing, mayonnaise-type, reduced-calorie	1 tbsp	Coffee whitener, powder	4 tsp
		Cream (light, coffee, table)	2 tbsp
Salad dressing, all varieties, regular	1 tbsp	Cream, sour	2 tbsp
		Cream (heavy, whipping)	1 tbsp
§Salad dressing, reduced-calorie (2 tbsp of low-calorie dressing is a free food)	2 tbsp	Cream cheese	1 tbsp
		*Salt pork	¼ oz

*400 mg or more of sodium if more than one or two servings are eaten

SATURATED FATS

Butter	1 tsp
*Bacon	1 slice

Free Foods

A free food is any food or drink that contains fewer than twenty calories per serving. You can eat as much as you want of items that have no serving size specified. You may eat two or three servings per day of those items that have a specific serving size. Be sure to spread them out through the day.

DRINKS	Carbonated water	Tonic water, sugar-free	Rhubarb, unsweetened (½ cup)
Bouillon § or broth without fat	Club soda		
	Cocoa powder, unsweetened (1 tbsp)	**NONSTICK PAN SPRAY**	
Bouillon, low-sodium			**VEGETABLES** (raw, 1 cup)
		FRUIT	
Carbonated drinks, sugar-free	Coffee/tea	Cranberries, unsweetened (½ cup)	Cabbage
	Drink mixes, sugar-free		Celery
			Chinese cabbage ¶

FREE FOODS (CONTINUED)

Cucumber

Green onion

Hot peppers

Mushrooms

Radishes

Zucchini ¶

SALAD GREENS

Endive

Escarole

Lettuce

Romaine

Spinach

SWEETS

Candy, hard, sugar-free

Gelatin, sugar-free

Gum, sugar-free

Jam/jelly, sugar-free (2 tsp)

Pancake syrup, sugar-free (1–2 tbsp)

Sugar substitutes (saccharin, aspartame)

Whipped topping (2 tbsp)

CONDIMENTS

Catsup (1 tbsp)

Horseradish

Mustard

Pickles §, dill, unsweetened

Salad dressing, low-calorie (2 tbsp)

Taco sauce (1 tbsp)

Vinegar

SEASONINGS

Seasonings can be very helpful in making foods taste better. Be careful of how much sodium you use. Read labels to help you choose seasonings that do not contain sodium or salt.

Basil (fresh)

Celery seeds

Cinnamon

Chili powder

Chives

Curry

Dill

Flavoring extracts (vanilla, almond, walnut, peppermint, butter, lemon, etc.)

Garlic

Garlic powder

Herbs

Hot pepper sauce

Lemon

Lemon juice

Lemon pepper

Lime

Lime juice

Mint

Onion powder

Oregano

Paprika

Pepper

Pimento

Spices

Soy sauce §

Soy sauce, low sodium ("lite")

Wine, used in cooking (¼ cup)

Worcestershire sauce

Combination Foods

Much of the food we eat is mixed together in various combinations. These combination foods do not fit into only one exchange list. It can be quite hard to tell what is in a certain casserole dish or baked food item. Following is a list of average values for some typical combination foods to help you fit these foods into your meal plan. Ask your dietitian for information about any other foods you'd like to eat. The American Diabetes Association/American Dietetic Association *Family Cookbooks* and the American Diabetes Association *Holiday Cookbook* have many recipes and further information about many foods, including combination foods. Check your library or local bookstore.

Food	Amount	Exchanges
Casserole, homemade	1 cup (8 oz)	2 medium-fat meat, 2 starches, 1 fat
Cheese pizza §, thin crust	¼ of a 15-oz size pizza or a 10″ pizza	1 medium-fat meat, 2 starches, 1 fat
Chili with beans ¶, § (commercial)	1 cup (8 oz)	2 medium-fat meat, 2 starches, 2 fats
Chow mein ¶, § (without noodles or rice)	2 cups (16 oz)	2 lean meat, 1 starch, 2 vegetable
Macaroni and cheese §	1 cup (8 oz)	1 medium-fat meat, 2 starches, 2 fats
Soup		
Bean ¶, §	1 cup (8 oz)	1 lean meat, 1 starch, 1 vegetable
Chunky, all varieties §	10¾-oz can	1 medium-fat meat, 1 starch, 1 vegetable
Cream § (made with water)	1 cup (8 oz)	1 starch, 1 fat
Vegetable § or broth §	1 cup (8 oz)	1 starch
Spaghetti and meatballs § (canned)	1 cup (8 oz)	1 medium-fat meat, 1 fat, 2 starches
Sugar-free pudding (made with skim milk)	½ cup	1 starch
If beans are used as a meat substitute:		
Dried beans ¶, peas ¶, lentils ¶	1 cup (cooked)	1 lean meat, 2 starches

Foods for Occasional Use

Moderate amounts of some foods can be used in your meal plan, in spite of their sugar or fat content, as long as you can maintain blood-glucose control. The following list includes average exchange values for some of these foods. Because they are concentrated sources of carbohydrate, you will notice that the portion sizes are very small. Check with your dietitian for advice on how often and when you can eat them.

Food	Amount	Exchanges
Angel-food cake	¹⁄₁₂ cake	2 starches
Cake, no icing	¹⁄₁₂ cake (3-in. square)	2 starches, 2 fats
Cookies	2 small (1¾ in. across)	2 starches, 1 fat
Frozen fruit yogurt	⅓ cup	1 starch
Gingersnaps	3	1 starch
Granola	¼ cup	1 starch, 1 fat
Granola bars	1 small	1 starch, 1 fat
Ice cream, any flavor	½ cup	1 starch, 2 fats
Ice milk, any flavor	½ cup	1 starch, 1 fat
Sherbet, any flavor	¼ cup	1 starch
*Snack chips, all varieties	1 oz	1 starch, 2 fats
Vanilla wafers	6 small	1 starch, 1 fat

*if more than one serving is eaten, these foods have 400 mg or more of sodium

Management Tips

Here are some tips that can help you to change the way you eat.

MAKE CHANGES GRADUALLY.   Don't try to do everything all at once. It may take longer to accomplish your goals, but the changes you make will be permanent.

SET SHORT-TERM, REALISTIC GOALS.   If weight loss is your goal, try to lose two pounds in two weeks, not twenty pounds in one week. Walk two blocks at first, not two miles. Success will come more easily, and you'll feel good about yourself.

REWARD YOURSELF.   When you achieve your short-term goal, do something special for yourself—go to a movie, buy a new shirt, read a book, visit a friend.

MEASURE FOODS.   It is important to eat the right serving sizes of food. You will need to learn how to estimate the amount of food you are served. You can do this by measuring all the food you eat for a week or so. Measure liquids with a measuring cup. Some solid foods (such as tuna, cottage cheese, and canned fruits) can also be measured with a measuring cup. Measuring spoons are used for measuring smaller amounts of other foods (such as oil, salad dressing, and peanut butter). A scale can be very useful for measuring almost anything, especially meat, poultry, and fish. All food should be measured or weighed after cooking.

Some food you buy uncooked will weigh less after you cook it. This is true of most meats. Starches often swell in cooking, so a small amount of uncooked starch will become a much larger amount of cooked food. The following table shows some of the changes:

Starch Group	Uncooked	Cooked
Oatmeal	3 level tbsp	½ cup
Cream of Wheat	2 level tbsp	½ cup
Grits	3 level tbsp	½ cup
Rice	2 level tbsp	⅓ cup
Spaghetti	¼ cup	½ cup
Noodles	⅓ cup	½ cup
Macaroni	¼ cup	½ cup
Dried beans	3 tbsp	⅓ cup
Dried peas	3 tbsp	⅓ cup
Lentils	2 tbsp	⅓ cup
Meat group		
Hamburger	4 oz	3 oz
Chicken	1 small drumstick	1 oz
	½ of a whole chicken breast	3 oz

READ FOOD LABELS.   Remember, *dietetic* does not mean *diabetic!* When you see the word "dietetic" on a food label, it means that something has been changed or replaced. It may have less salt, less fat, or less sugar. It does *not* mean that the food is sugar-free or calorie-free. Some dietetic foods may be useful. Those that contain twenty calories or less per serving may be eaten up to three times a day as free foods.

KNOW YOUR SWEETENERS.   Two types of sweeteners are on the market: those with calories, and those without calories. Sweeteners with calories (such as fructose, sorbitol, and mannitol) may cause cramping and diarrhea when used in large amounts. Remember, these sweeteners *do* have calories, which can add up. Sweeteners without calories include saccharin and aspartame (Equal, Nutrasweet) and may be used in moderation.

If You Have Insulin-Dependent Diabetes

PLAN FOR SICK DAYS.   *Before* you become ill with the flu or a cold, ask your doctor, dietitian, or nurse for a special sick-day plan. When you are ill, it is important to do the following:

Take your usual insulin dose.

Test your blood glucose regularly, and check your urine for ketones.

If you can't keep regular food down, try drinking small sips of regular soft drinks, sweetened tea, sweetened gelatin, Popsicles, fruit juice, or sherbet. (Call your doctor immediately if you can't keep any food down.)

Drink lots of liquids.

PREPARE FOR INSULIN REACTIONS.   If you have symptoms of low blood glucose, test your blood to find out your blood-glucose level. Be sure to carry something with you at all times to treat low blood glucose (for example, glucose tablets or hard candy).

PLAN FOR EXERCISE.   You may need to make some changes in your meal plan or insulin dose when you begin an exercise program. Check with your dietitian or doctor about this. Be sure to carry some form of carbohydrate with you to treat low blood glucose (for example, dried fruit or glucose tablets). Additional information on these topics is available from your dietitian or doctor.

Glossary

Alcohol   An ingredient in a variety of beverages, including beer, wine, liqueurs, cordials, and mixed or straight drinks. Pure alcohol itself yields about seven calories per gram, of which more than 75 percent is available to the body.

Calorie   A unit used to express the energy value of food. Calories come from carbohydrates, proteins, fats, and alcohol.

Carbohydrate   One of the three major energy sources in foods. The most common carbohydrates are sugar and starches. Carbohydrates yield about four calories per gram. Carbohydrates are found in foods from the milk, vegetable, fruit, and starch/bread exchange lists.

Cholesterol   A fatlike substance normally found in blood. A high level of cholesterol in the blood has been shown to be a major risk factor for developing heart disease. Dietary cholesterol is found in all animal products, but it is especially high in egg yolks and organ meats. Eating foods high in dietary cholesterol and saturated fat tends to raise the level of blood cholesterol. Foods of plant origin, such as fruits, vegetables, grains, and legumes, contain no cholesterol. Cholesterol is found in foods from the milk, meat, and fat exchange lists.

Dietitian   A registered dietitian (R.D.) is recognized by the medical profession as the primary provider of nutritional care, education, and counseling. The initials "R.D." after a dietitian's name ensure that he or she has met the standards of the American Dietetic Association. Look for this credential when you seek advice on nutrition.

Exchange   Foods grouped together on a list according to similarities in food values. Measured amounts of foods within the group may be used as trade-offs in planning meals. All of the exchanges in a group contain approximately equal amounts of carbohydrate, protein, fat, and calories.

Fat   One of the three energy sources in food. A concentrated source of calories, with about nine calories per gram. Fat is found in foods from the fat and meat exchange lists. Some kinds of milk also have fat, as do some foods from the starch/bread list.

Saturated fat   This fat tends to raise blood-cholesterol levels. It comes primarily from animals and is often hard at room temperature. Examples of saturated fats are butter, lard, meat fat, solid shortening, palm oil, and coconut oil.

Unsaturated fat This type of fat—monounsaturated in particular—tends to lower blood-cholesterol levels. Polyunsaturated fat neither raises nor lowers them. Unsaturated fat comes from plants and is usually liquid at room temperature. Examples of monounsaturated fats are olive, canola, and avocado oils, while examples of polyunsaturated fats are corn, cottonseed, sunflower, safflower, and soybean oils.

Fiber An indigestible part of certain foods. Fiber is important in the diet as roughage, or bulk. Fiber is found in foods from the starch/bread, vegetable, and fruit exchange lists.

Soluble fiber Has high water-holding capability and turns to gel during digestion, which slows digestion and the rate of nutrition absorption from the stomach and intestine. This type of fiber is found in oat bran, pectins (in fruits and vegetables), and various "gums" that are found in nuts, seeds, and legumes such as beans, lentils, and peas. This type of fiber may play a role in smoothing out the glycemic response of foods and in reducing the likelihood of arteriosclerosis.

Insoluble fiber Found in foods such as wheat bran and other whole grains; has poor water-holding capability. It appears to speed the passage of foods through the stomach and intestines, and it increases fecal bulk. This type of fiber probably does not affect glycemic response or arteriosclerosis.

Glycosylated hemoglobin A test that gives information about blood-glucose levels during the preceding one to two months. When blood glucose is above normal, the glucose changes the hemoglobin in red blood cells. These cells last for about 100 days and can be measured.

Gram A unit of mass and weight in the metric system. One ounce is equal to about 30 grams.

IDDM Insulin-dependent diabetes mellitus. Individuals with IDDM are ketosis-prone and will develop ketoacidosis if they do not take insulin regularly.

Insulin A hormone made by the body that helps the body use food. Also, a commercially prepared injectable substance used by people who do not make enough of their own insulin.

Ketoacidosis An increase in ketones in the blood, causing the body's acid balance to tip. An emergency situation that may result in coma and death if untreated.

Ketone   An acid that forms in the body when fats are burned for energy.

Meal plan   A guide showing the number of food exchanges to use in each meal and snack to control the distribution of carbohydrates, proteins, fats, and calories throughout the day.

Mineral   Substance essential in small amounts to build and repair body tissue and/or control functions of the body. Examples include calcium, iron, magnesium, phosphorus, potassium, sodium, and zinc.

NIDDM   Non–insulin-dependent diabetes mellitus. Individuals with NIDDM may or may not need to take insulin for better control of their blood-glucose levels; however, they are not ketosis-prone.

Nutrient   Substance in food necessary for life. Carbohydrates, protein, fats, minerals, vitamins, and water are nutrients.

Nutrition   Combination of processes by which the body receives and uses the materials necessary for maintenance of functions, for energy, and for growth and renewal of its parts.

Protein   One of the three major nutrients in food. Protein provides about four calories per gram. Protein is found in foods from the milk and meat exchange lists. Smaller amounts of protein are found in foods from the vegetable and starch/bread lists.

Sodium   A mineral needed by the body to maintain life, found mainly as a component of salt. Many individuals need to cut down the amount of sodium (and salt) they eat to help control high blood pressure.

Starch   One of the two major types of carbohydrates. Foods consisting mainly of starch come from the starch/bread exchange list.

Sugar   One of the two major types of carbohydrates. Foods consisting mainly of simple sugars are those from the milk, vegetable, and fruit exchange lists. Other simple sugars include common table sugar and the sugar alcohols (sorbitol, mannitol, etc.)

Triglycerides   A fat that the body makes from food and that is normally present in the blood. Excess weight or consumption of too much fat, alcohol, and sugar may increase the blood triglycerides to an unacceptably high level.

Vitamins   Substances found in food and needed in small amounts to assist in bodily processes and functions. These include vitamins A, D, E, B-complex, C, and K.

Appendix D

Points in Nutrition

Food Choices

Menu items	Calorie points*	Menu items	Calorie points*
Apple, 1–3" diam	1	Butter, 1 pat	½
Applesauce, ½ c	1	Cabbage, ½ c	0
Apricots, 3 halves	½	Cantaloupe, 1 c	1
Asparagus, ½ c	½	Carrot, ½	0
Avocado, ½–3" diam	2	Casserole, 1 c	5
Bacon, 1 slice	½	Cauliflower, ½ c	0
Bagel, 1–3" diam	2	Cottage cheese	
Banana, 1–9"	1½	4% fat, ½ c	1½
Beans		Cheese	
*baked, ½ c	2	hard yellow, 1 oz	1½
navy, ½ c	1½	Chicken, 1 oz	1
green, ½ c	0	Cold cuts, 1 slice	1
Beef, lean, 1 oz	1	Corn, ½ c	1
Beef stew, 1 c	3	Corn bread, 2" square	2½
Beer		Corn flakes, 1 c	1½
regular, 12 oz	2	Crackers, 3 sq	½
lite, 12 oz	1½	(standard-size saltine crackers)	
Biscuit, 2" diam	1½	Cream	
Bran, 100%, ½ c	1½	half and half, 2 tbsp	½
Bran flakes, ½ c	1½	sour cream, 2 tbsp	½
Bread, 1 slice	1	Croissant, 1	3
Broccoli, ⅔ c	½	Egg, 1	1
Brussels sprouts, 7–8	½	Fat (margarine, oil)	
Buns		1 tsp.	½
hamburger or hot dog	1½	Fish, 2 oz	1
		Grapes, 1 c	1

*75 calories = 1 point

178

Menu items	Calorie points*
Grapefruit	
Fresh, ½	½
Juice, 1 c	1
Grape juice, 1 c	2
Lamb, lean, 2 oz	1½
Macaroni, 1 c	2
Mayonnaise, 1 tbsp	1½
Milk	
2%, 1 c	1½
skim, 1 c	1
whole, 1 c	2
Muffin, 3″ diam	1½
Noodles, 1 c	3
Nuts	
cashews, 6–8	1
mixed, 8–12	1
walnuts, 8–10	1
Oatmeal, 1 c	2
Oils, 1 tbsp	1½
Olives, 6	½
Onions, ½ c	½
Orange, 3″	1
Orange juice, 1 c	1½
Pancake, 6″ diam	2
Peach, 3″ diam	½
Peanuts, 1 oz	2
Peanut butter, 2 tsp	1
Pear, 3 x 4″	1½
Peas, green, ½ c	1
Pepper, green, 1 large	½
Pineapple (unsweetened)	
canned, 1 c	2
juice, 1 c	2

Menu items	Calorie points*
Pita bread, 6″ diam	2
Plums, 1 medium	½
Popcorn, plain, 3 c	1
Pork, lean, 1 oz	1
Potatoes	
baked, 1 medium	2
chips, 2 oz	4
french-fried, ten 4″ strips	2
hash browns, ½ c	2½
mashed, ½ c	1½
Pretzels, 6 sticks	1
Prunes	
canned, 5	1
juice, 1 c	2½
Raisins, 2 tbsp	½
Rice, 1 c	3
Roll, 2″ diam	1
Salad dressing, 1 tbsp	1
Sauerkraut, ½ c	½
Spaghetti, 1 c	2
Spinach, 1 c	½
Squash, winter, ½ c	½
Strawberries, 1 c	½
Sweet potato, 2 x 4″	3
Tomato	
raw, 1 medium	½
juice, 1 c	½
*catsup, 2 tbsp	½
Veal, 2 oz	2
Waffle, 7″ diam	3½
Watermelon, 1 c	½
Yogurt, plain, 1 c	2

*Contains sugar.

Free Foods:
Lettuce, greens, small amounts of raw vegetables, beverages with 0 calories

Decaffeinated beverages are preferred. Fruits are unsweetened. Vegetables have no added fat. Meats are baked or broiled.

c = cup; diam = diameter
oz = ounce; sq = square
tbsp = tablespoon;
tsp = teaspoon
" = inch

This is not a complete index of points or portion sizes.

For more information, consult:
"Points in Your Favor"
St. Joseph Medical Center
Dietary Department
3600 E. Harry
Wichita, KS 67218

Appendix E

Restaurant Guide

Food Choices

Menu items	Calorie points†
ARBY's	
Arby's Sauce, 1 oz	½
Arby's Sub (no dressing)	6½
Bac 'n' Cheddar Deluxe	7½
Beef 'n' Cheddar	6½
Chicken Breast Sandwich	8
Chicken Club Sandwich	8½
Chicken Salad Croissant	6
French Dip	5
French Fries (2½ oz)	4
Ham 'n' Cheese	6½
Horsey Sauce, 1 oz	½
Potato	
Broccoli & Cheese	7½
Deluxe	9
Mushroom & Cheese	7
Taco	8½
Potato Cakes, 2	2½
Roast Beef	
Deluxe	6½
Junior	3
Regular	4½
Super	8½
Roasted Chicken	3½
Shake	
*Chocolate, small	5

Menu items	Calorie points
*Jamocha, small	5½
*Vanilla, small	4½
Breakfast	
Croissant	
Arby's Butter	3
Bacon & Egg	5½
Ham & Swiss	4½
Mushroom & Swiss	4½
Sausage & Egg	7
BRAUM's	
Hamburger	6
Cheeseburger	5
Steak Sandwich	8½
French Fries, large order	5
small	2½
*Ice Cream Cone, one dip	2½
BURGER KING	
Bacon Double Cheeseburger	8
Cheeseburger	5
Double	7
French Fries, regular	3
Hamburger	4
Double	5½
Onion Rings, regular	3½

*Contains too much sugar.
†75 calories = 1 pt

Menu items	Calorie points
Specialty Chicken Sandwich	9½
Specialty Ham & Cheese Sandwich	7½
Whaler Sandwich	7½
Whaler Sandwich with Cheese	8
Whopper Jr.	5
Whopper Jr. with Cheese	5½
Whopper	9
Double	12
Whopper with Cheese	10
Double	13
Veal Parmigiana	8

Breakfast

Croissanwich	
Plain	3
With Egg	4½
With Cheese	4½
With Egg & Cheese	6
and Sausage	8½
and Bacon	7

CHURCH's FRIED CHICKEN

1 Piece Chicken	4
2 Large Pieces with Dinner Roll	9
3 Large Pieces with Dinner Roll	13
Dinner Roll	1
French Fries	3½
Corn on the Cob	2
Fried Okra	3
Coleslaw	1

Menu items	Calorie points
DAIRY QUEEN	
Cheeseburger	5½
Double	9
Triple	11
Chicken Sandwich	9
*Ice Cream Cone, small	2
*Ice Cream Cone, regular	3
*Ice Cream Cone, large	4½
Dilly Bar	3
Fish Sandwich	5½
with Cheese	6
French Fries	
regular	2½
large	4½
Hamburger	5
Double	7
Triple	9½
Hot Dog	4
Hot Dog with Cheese	4½
Hot Dog with Chili	4½
Onion Rings, regular	4
Super Hot Dog	7
with Cheese	8
with Chili	8

DENNY's

Denny's Combo (hamburger, fries, and salad or soup)	12
Low-Calorie Plate	6
Chicken Salad Plate	6½
Beef-adelphia	11½
Chicken Fried Steak	8
Fried Chicken	13

---

*Contains too much sugar.

Menu items	Calorie points
GODFATHER'S PIZZA	
Pizza, ½ of small pizza	
Beef	7
Pepperoni	7½
Sausage	8
Combination	9½
Ham and Cheese Sandwich	7½
Supreme Sandwich	9
GRANDY's	
Scrambled Eggs with Hash Browns, Biscuit, Gravy	
with Sausage	12
with Bacon	9½
with Breakfast Steak	13½
Hotcakes	
with Sausage	6½
with Bacon	4
with Breakfast Steak	8
Hot Biscuit Sandwich	
with Sausage	6
with Bacon	4
with Egg and Cheese	6
One Biscuit and Gravy	4
*"Sinnamon" Roll	5
*Syrup, 1 tbsp	1
BBQ Ribs	
Coleslaw or Beans, BBQ Sauce, Roll	
and 2 Ribs	11
and 3 Ribs	14
Country Fried Steak, Potatoes, Gravy, Coleslaw or Beans, and 2 rolls	9½

*Contains too much sugar.

Menu items	Calorie points
Fried Chicken	
1 Piece Chicken, Vegetable, and Roll	5
2 Pieces of Chicken, Coleslaw or Beans, and Roll	8½
Baked Beans	2
Coleslaw	1
French Fries	4
GRINDER MAN	
Mini: Peppered Beef, Roast Beef, Canadian Bacon, Italian Style Ham, Sausage, or Ham	6
Mini: Meatball, Club, Turkey, Pepperoni & Provolone, or Pepperoni & Mozzarella	5½
Mini: Vegetarian, or Provolone & Sauce	5
Mini: Reuben, Mozzarella & Sauce, or Ham/Rye	4½
Mini: Pastrami	6½
Mini: Grinder	7
Mini: Hero	7½
Mini: Sicilian Red or Genoa	8
Mini: Copoccolo, Black or Red	8½
HARDEE's	
Breakfast	
Biscuit	3½
Bacon & Egg	5½
Egg	5
Gravy	5½
Ham	4½
Ham & Egg	6
Sausage	5½
Sausage & Egg	7

Menu items	Calorie points
Steak	5½
Steak & Egg	7
Fried Egg	1½
Hash Rounds	2½
Other Items	
*Apple Turnover	4
Bacon Cheeseburger	9½
*Big Cookie	4
Big Deluxe	7½
Big Roast Beef	5½
Cheeseburger	4½
Chef Salad	3½
Chicken Fillet	7
Fisherman's Fillet	6½
French Fries, small	3
French Fries, large	5
Hamburger	4
Hot Dog	4½
Hot Ham 'n' Cheese	5
Mushroom 'n' Swiss	7
Roast Beef Sandwich	5
Shrimp Salad	5
Turkey Club	6

KENTUCKY FRIED CHICKEN

Menu items	Calorie points
Chicken Breast Sandwich	6
Coleslaw, ¾ c	1½
Corn, 5½" ear	2½
Extra-Crispy Chicken	
Drumstick	2
Keel	4
Side Breast	4
Thigh	4½
Wing	2½

Menu items	Calorie points
Extra-Crispy Dinner (includes Mashed Potatoes, Gravy, Coleslaw, Roll) and	
Drumstick & Thigh	10½
Wing & Side Breast	10
Wing & Thigh	12
Gravy, 1 tbsp	½
Kentucky Fries (3.4 oz)	2½
Mashed Potatoes (3 oz)	1
Original Recipe Chicken	
Drumstick	1½
Keel	3
Side Breast	2½
Thigh	3½
Wing	2
Original Recipe Dinner (includes Mashed Potatoes, Gravy, Coleslaw, Roll) and	
Drumstick & Thigh	8½
Wing & Side Breast	8
Wing & Thigh	9
Roll	1

LONG JOHN SILVER'S SEAFOOD SHOPPE

Menu items	Calorie points
Chicken Planks	6
Clam Dinner (6 oz Clams, 3 oz Fries, 4 oz Coleslaw)	12
Coleslaw, 4 oz	2
Corn on the Cob, 1 ear	2½
Fish, 1 piece	2½
Fish, 2 pieces	5
Fish, 3 pieces	7½
Fish & Chicken Dinner (1 Fish, 2 Chicken Planks, 3 oz Fries, 4 oz Coleslaw)	11½

*Contains too much sugar.

Menu items	Calorie points
Fish & Fries	
(3 Fish, 3 oz Fries)	11½
Fish & More (2 Fish, 2 Hush Puppies, 3 oz Fries, 4 oz Coleslaw)	12
French Fries (3 oz)	4
Hush Puppies	1½
Oyster Dinner (6 Oysters, 3 oz Fries, 4 oz Coleslaw)	11
Peg Legs, 5	6
Scallop Dinner (6 Scallops, 3 oz Fries, 4 oz Coleslaw)	9½
Seafood Platter (1 Fish, 2 Scallops, 2 Shrimp, 2 Hush Puppies, 3 oz Fries, 4 oz Coleslaw)	12
Shrimp, 6 Pieces	3½
Treasure Chest (2 Fish, 2 Peg Legs, 3 oz Fries, 4 oz Coleslaw)	13

LONGNECKER's

Hamburger II	6
"The Hamburger"	8
Hot Dog, plain	7
Fries	5
Steak Sandwich	7

McDONALD's
Breakfast
Biscuits

Bacon, Egg, and Cheese	6½
Biscuit Only	4½
Sausage	6½
Sausage and Egg	8
English Muffin with Butter	2½

Menu items	Calorie points
Hash Brown Potatoes (½ c)	1½
McMuffins	
Egg	4½
Sausage	6
Sausage with Eggs	7
Sausage (2)	3
Scrambled Eggs	2½
Other Items	
*Apple Pie	3½
Big Mac	7½
Cheeseburger	4½
Chicken McNuggets 6 Pieces	4½
*BBQ Sauce	1
*Honey Sauce	½
Hot Mustard Sauce	1
*Sweet-Sour Sauce	1
*Chocolate-Chip Cookies	4½
*Ice Cream Cone	2½
Filet-o-Fish	6
French Fries, regular	3
Hamburger	3½
McD.L.T.	8
*McDonaldland Cookies	4
McPizza	4½
Quarter Pounder	6
Quarter Pounder with Cheese	7

ORIENTAL FOOD ESTIMATES

Almond Chicken	7
Broccoli Beef, 1½ c	6
Chinese Noodles, 1 c	4
Chop Suey, 1 c, any meat	3
Chow Mein, 1 c, any meat	3

*Contains too much sugar.

Menu items	Calorie points
Egg Roll, 4″	3
Fried Rice, 1 c	4
Moo Goo Gai Pan	6
Rice, 1 c	3

PIZZA HUT**
Pan Pizza (2 slices)

Cheese	8½
Pepperoni	9
Supreme	9½
Super Supreme	9

Priazzo Italian Pie (2 slices)

Roma	8
Milano	7½

Thin and Crispy Pizza (2 slices)

Cheese	6
Pepperoni	6½
Supreme	8½
Super Supreme	8

Personal Pan Pizza (whole)

Pepperoni, whole	8
Supreme, whole	9

Calizza

5-Cheese, whole	8½
Italian Sausage, whole	9

**based on a medium, 10″ pizza

RAX

Barbecue Beef Sandwich	4½
Beef, Bacon & Cheddar Sandwich	9
Big Rax Roast Beef	7½
Chicken Noodle Soup	2
Chicken Sandwich	8
*Chocolate-Chip Cookie	2

Menu items	Calorie points
Chowder	2½
French Fries	4½
Ham 'n' Cheese Sandwich	4½
Philly Beef 'n' Cheese Sandwich	7

Baked Potato

Plain	3½
Bacon & Cheese	8
Beef Barbecue	9½
Beef Stroganoff	7½
Broccoli & Cheese	7½
Margarine	5½
Mexican	8
Pizza	6½
Sour Cream	4½

Potato Skins

Bacon & Cheese Single	1½
Rax Roast Beef	5
Turkey Bacon Club Sandwich	7½
Vegetable Soup	1

RED LOBSTER
(Fish baked unless otherwise noted)

Albacore Tuna (3½ oz)	2
Breaded Fried Pollock (3½ oz)	2½
Breaded Fried Whiting (3½ oz)	2½
Broiled Fisherman's Platter	13
Broiled Stuffed Flounder Dinner	14
Clams (3½ oz)	1
Flounder (3½ oz)	1
Freshwater Catfish	1½

---

*Contains too much sugar.

Menu items	Calorie points
Fried Chicken, 4 pieces	6
Garlic Bread, 1 slice	2
Grouper (3½ oz)	1
Haddock (3½ oz)	1
Halibut (3½ oz)	1
Hamburger (3 oz)	3½
Hush Puppies (2)	2½
Lobster (3½ oz)	1½
Mariner's Platter	13
Oysters (3½ oz)	1
Perch (3½ oz)	1
Pollock (3½ oz)	1
Potato	1
Sample Platter	11
Scallops, steamed (3½ oz)	1
Shore Platter	11
Shrimp, boiled (3½ oz)	1
Sirloin Steak (3½ oz)	4½
Snapper (3½ oz)	1½
Snow Crab, boiled (3½ oz)	1
Sole (3½ oz)	1
Steak & Lobster Dinner	21
Tuna (3½ oz)	1½
Turbot (3½ oz)	1
Whiting (3½ oz)	1½

SCHLOTSKY's

Original, small	4
Original, medium	8
Original, large	16
Roast Sandwich	
medium	4½
large	5½

Menu items	Calorie points
Turkey Sandwich, medium	4
Turkey Sandwich, large	5

SONIC

Hamburger	6
Cheeseburger	7½
Steak Sandwich	8½
Fish Sandwich	5½
Corn Dog	6
Coney	7½
Chili Pie	6½
French Fries	4
Onion Rings	5
*Twist on Cone	4

SPANGLES

*Apple Pie	6
BBQ Chicken Sandwich	7
BBQ Ham Sandwich	4
BLT Burger (¼ lb)	7
Chicken Club	14
Chicken Sandwich	13
Chili Dog	9
Chili Frito Dish	13
Chili with Beans	
small	3½
large	7
Corn Dog	4½
Corn Dog with Cheese	5
French Fries, small	3
French Fries, large	5
Hamburger	5½
Triple	11½

*Contains too much sugar.

Menu items	Calorie points
Hickory Bacon	
Burger (¼ lb)	6½
Double (½ lb)	9½
Hot Dog	9
Kraut Dog	8½
Onion Rings	9
Polish Sausage	9½
Potato	
Bacon & Cheese	7½
BBQ Beef & Cheese	9½
Broccoli & Cheese	7½
Cheese	8
Chili & Cheese	8½
Sour Cream & Chives	7
Shredded Ham Sandwich	4

STEAK AND ALE

Menu items	Calorie points
French Onion Soup	3½
Dinner Entrees	
Beef and Shrimp Kabob	5
Kensington Club	8
Petit Filet,	
trimmed (6 oz)	4½
Broiled Shrimp Pilaf	
with Rice	6
Stuffed Flounder	
Maitre D'	6
Lobster Catch	4
Alaskan King Crab Feast	5
Drawn Butter (1 tbsp)	1½
Prime Rib, trimmed (8 oz)	6
Hawaiian Chicken (one breast)	
with Rice	5½

Menu items	Calorie points
SUB AND STUFF**	
Ham & Cheese	5½
Tuna	7
Sub Special	5½
Roast Beef	5
Sub & Stuff	6½
Turkey	5

**6-inch sandwiches made with onion, lettuce, tomato, green pepper, and black olives on white or wheat bread

TACO BELL

Menu items	Calorie points
Bean Burrito	4½
Beef Burrito	6½
Beefy Tostada	4
Bellbeefer	3
Bellbeefer with Cheese	4
Burrito Supreme	6
Combination Burrito	5½
Enchirito	6
Taco	2½
Taco Supreme	3½
Taco Salad	7½
Tostado, regular	2½
Bean Burrito	4
Combination Burrito	5½
Enchilada	4
Refried Beans	3
Sancho	5
Soft Taco	2½
Taco	5
Taco Burger	2½
Taco Dinner (taco, enchilada, beans, chips)	9½

Menu items	Calorie points
Tostado	2½
VILLAGE INN	
Egg, one	1½
Eggs, two	2½
Pancakes, three	3
Hash Browns	3
Bacon	2
Sausage	6
Ham	3
Toast	3
English Muffin	3
French Toast	7½
Omelettes	
Cheese	7
Three Egg	4½
Ham and Cheese	8
Western	6

Breakfast
Robert E. Lee: Buttermilk
Biscuits, Country Gravy, and
Hash Browns — 10

Eggs Benedict: Toasted English
Muffin topped with Canadian-
Style Bacon, 2 Poached Eggs,
and Hollandaise with Hash
Browns — 10

WENDY's
Breakfast

Bacon, 2 strips	1½
Breakfast Sandwich	5
*Danish, 1 piece	5
French Toast, 2 slices	5½
Home Fries	5

*Contains too much sugar.

Menu items	Calorie points
Omelette	
Ham & Cheese	3½
Ham, Cheese, & Mushroom	4
Ham, Cheese, Onion, & Green Pepper	4
Mushroom, Onion, & Green Pepper	3
Sausage, 1 pattie	2½
Scrambled Eggs	2½
Toast with Margarine, 2 slices	3½
Other Items	
Cheeseburger	6½
Double	9
Chicken Sandwich	4½
Chili (8 oz)	3½
French Fries, regular	4
*Frosty Dairy Dessert (12 oz)	5½
Salad Bar	
Breadstick	½
Cheese, Imitation (1 oz)	
American	1
Cheddar	1
Mozzarella	1
Swiss	1
Dressings (1 tbsp)	
Blue Cheese	1
Celery Seed	1
Golden Italian	½
Ranch	1
Red French	1
Thousand Island	1
Reduced-Calorie Dressing (1 tbsp)	
Bacon & Tomato	½
Creamy Cucumber	½

Menu items	Calorie points
Italian	½
Thousand Island	½
Sunflower Seeds and Raisins (¼ c)	2½
Hamburger	5
Double	8
Hot Stuffed Baked Potato (plain)	3½
with	
Bacon & Cheese	7½
Broccoli & Cheese	7
Cheese	8
Chicken à la King	4½
Sour Cream & Chives	6
Stroganoff & Sour Cream	6½
Pasta Salad (½ c)	2
Side Salad	1½
Taco Salad	5½

WHITE CASTLE

Cheeseburger	2½
Fish Sandwich	2½
French Fries	3
Hamburger	2

YOGURT HEAVEN

*Frozen Yogurt (4 oz)	2
*Tofree (4 oz)	1½

SALAD BAR INGREDIENTS

#Bean Sprouts, ⅓ c	0
#Beets, ¼ c	0
#Bell Pepper, ¼ c	0
# Cabbage, Red, ½ c	0
# Carrot, ½	0

Menu items	Calorie points
# Cauliflower, ¼ c	0
Cheese, American, 2 tbsp	1½
Coleslaw, ½ c	1
Cottage Cheese, ⅓ c	1
Croutons, ¼ c	1
# Cucumber, 4 slices	0
Eggs, chopped, ¼ c	1
Kidney beans, ⅓ c	1
#Lettuce, chopped, 2 c	0
#Mushrooms, fresh, ¼ c	0
Potato Salad, ½ c	2½
#Radishes, ¼ c	0
Raisins, 2 tbsp	½
#Red Onions, ¼ c	0
#Spring Onions, 2 medium	0
Sunflower Seeds, 1 tbsp	1
#Tomatoes, Cherry, 3 medium	0
#Choice of any three	½

Salad Dressing (1 tbsp)

Blue Cheese	1
Celery Seed	1
Golden Italian	1
Ranch	1
Red French	1
Thousand Island	1

Reduced-Calorie Salad Dressing (1 tbsp)

Bacon & Tomato	½
Creamy Cucumber	½
Italian	½
Thousand Island	½
Wine Vinegar	0

*Contains too much sugar.

Menu items	Calorie points	Menu items	Calorie points
Soft Drinks (12 oz)		*Pepsi Cola	2
*Coca-Cola	2	Diet Pepsi	0
Diet Coke	0	*Root Beer	2
*Orange Drink	2	*Sprite	2

*Contains too much sugar.

Appendix F

Metabolic (MET) Levels of Activities

Definitions

MET—The metabolic rate refers to oxygen consumption. (Note: Values do not refer to duration of effort or total expenditure over some period of time.)

Static tension (+) = Static, or isometric, component of an activity that increases the work required of the heart.

Points to consider before initiating specific tasks:

1. MET level at which you are functioning.
2. Environment: temperature, clothing, emotional stress, position.
3. Duration: you should have full recovery without fatigue within an hour of activity.

Calculation of METs:

Duration of activity (in hours or portions of hours) × MET number = subtotal of METs. Sum of subtotal of METs = total METs. (Average adult is expected to accumulate 30–40 METs/day.)

Activities Listed by MET Levels

Self-care METs

Sitting in a chair	1.0
Care for fingernails	1.2
Brush teeth	1.2
Eating a meal	1.3
Wash hands and face	1.5
Wash upper body	1.5

Baths in tub	1.5
Comb hair, male and female	1.5
Sit on edge of bed	1.5
Sit on bedside commode	1.5
Shave, electric and safety razor	1.6
Wash hair, male and female	1.5+
Set hair	1.6+
Wash entire body sitting in bathroom	1.7+
Shower, sit	1.8+
Dress and undress nightclothes	2.0+
Dress and undress street clothes	2.0+
Shower, stand	3.8
Use bedpan	4.8

Housework

Machine sewing, household	2.3
Washing small clothes	2.5
Mix batter	2.5+
Peel potatoes	3.2
Fix simple meal (breakfast or lunch)	2–3.0
Fold clothes	2–3+
Wash clothes (by machine)	2.3+
Fix complex meal (dinner)	3+
Wash dishes	3+
Ironing, standing	3++
Scrubbing at counter height, standing	3++
Making bed	2–3++
Bending and stooping (picking up newspaper)	3++
Cleaning stove (inside)	3–4++
Scrub pots and pans	3–4++
Dusting/polishing (reaching with arms)	3–4++
Changing bed	3–4++
Wringing by hand	4.5
Hanging wash	4.6

Mopping floors (hands and knees)	3–5++
Vacuuming (bare floor to pile rugs)	4–5++
Sweeping floor	4–5++
Mopping (standing)	4–5++
Grocery shopping	4–5++++
Scrubbing, polishing, waxing floors, walls, cars, windows while standing	5–6+++
Turning mattress	7+++++

Vocational

Sitting at desk, writing, calculating	1.5
Lying down under a car to do repair	1.5
Using hand tools	1.8
Light assembly work	1.8
Radio repair	1.8
Driving a truck	1.8
Working heavy levers	2
Dredge	2
Watch repairing	2.1
Bookbinding, light	2.3
Typing rapidly	2.3
Power sanding or sawing	2.6
Armature winding	2.6
Bricklaying	3–5+++
Plastering	3–5+++
Carpentry	4–6++++
Lift maximum 50 lb; frequently lift/carry 25 lb	4–6++++
Pushing wheelbarrow, 50 lb	4++++
Shoveling	5–7++++
Digging holes	5–7++++
Chopping wood	5–7++++
Light/heavy farming	5–7+++
Light/heavy industrial	5–7+++
Lift maximum 100 lb; frequently lift/carry 50 lb	6–8+++++

Avocational/Recreational

Phoning, conversation	1.0
Leather punching, lacing, back supported	1.8
Leather tooling, back supported	1.8
Making link belt, back supported	1.9
Rug hooking, sitting	1.9
Hand sewing	2
Knitting, 23 stitches/minute	2
Embroidery	2
Playing cards or any sitting competitive game	2
Chip carving, back supported	2.1
Copper tooling	2.2
Weaving, table loom	2.2
Leather carving, sitting	2.3
Painting, sitting	2.5
Chisel carving with mallet, sitting	2.5
Printing (hand composition)	2.6
Horsehoes	3
Horseback riding, walk	3.3
Playing organ, sitting	3.5
Playing piano	2–3++
Hammering	3++++
Walking, 2.5 mph	3+
Lift 20 lb maximum; frequently lift 10 lb	3.5+++
Volleyball	3.8
Planting	3–4
Riding motorcycle	3–4+++
Painting wall	3–4++
Cycling, 5.5 mph	3–4++
Sexual activity	3–4+++
Playing drums	4.3
Bowling	4.5
Gardening	4.7
Badminton	4.5

Ping-Pong	4–5
Archery	4–5
Walking down stairs	4.5
Swimming, breast stroke, 20 yd/min	5
Weeding	3–5+
Sailing	2–5+
Walking, 3.5 mph	5.5+
Hoeing	4–6++
Canoeing, 2–5 mph	3–6+++
Golfing	4–7
Hunting	4–6
Sawing wood	5–7
Ice skating	5–7
Horseback riding, trotting	7.5
Mowing lawn by hand or power	8
Dancing, fox-trot	5–7+++
Spading	3–8
Cycling, 13 mph	7–9
Skiing (snow or water)	9
Squash	9
Tennis	5–15+

Appendix G

Some Calorie/Exercise Expenditures

The following are lists of various classifications of work and recreation in relation to calories expended per minute.

Work	Calories/min
Light	2.5
Moderate	5.0
Heavy	7.5
Very heavy	10.0
Extremely heavy	12.5
Rest	1.25

Locomotion	
Wheelchair, 1.2 mph	2.4
Walking, 2.5 mph	3.6
Walking, 2.75 mph	5.6
Walking down stairs	5.2
Walking with crutches and/or braces, 1.2 mph	8.0
Walking up stairs, (17-lb load, 27 ft/min)	9.0
Walking up stairs (no load)	8.0

Exercises	
Bending at waist (sideways), 13/min	2.2
Sitting on floor, touching toes, 16/min	2.4
Balancing exercises	2.5
Abdominal exercises	3.0
Lying on floor, leg raising, 10/min	3.5
Trunk bending	3.5

| Arm swinging, hopping | 6.5 |
| Push-ups, 16/min | 7.5 |

Self-care

Resting, supine	1.0
Sitting	1.2
Standing, relaxed	1.4
Eating	1.4
Conversing	1.4
Dressing, undressing	2.3
Washing hands, face, brushing hair	2.5
Washing and shaving	2.6
Washing and dressing	2.6
Using bedside commode	3.6
Showering	4.2
Using a bedpan	4.7

Household tasks

Hand sewing	1.4
Knitting	1.5
Sweeping	1.7
Ironing, standing	1.7
Machine sewing	1.8
Simple work, sitting	1.7
Brushing boots	2.2
Polishing	2.4
Peeling potatoes	2.9
Scrubbing, standing	2.9
Washing small clothes	3.0
Bringing in wash	3.3
Kneading dough	3.3
Scrubbing floors	3.6
Making beds	3.9
Cleaning windows	3.7
Mopping	4.2

Wringing by hand	4.4
Hanging wash	4.5
Polishing floors	4.8
Beating carpets	4.9
Breaking firewood	4.9
Making and stripping bed	5.4
Clearing floors, kneeling, bending	6.0

Children's Recreation

Sitting, listening to radio	1.0
Sitting, playing with puzzle	1.2
Sitting, singing	1.4
Standing, drawing	1.5–1.9
Cycling	2.4–3.1
Carpentry	3.0

Recreation

Sitting, listening to radio	2.0–2.5
Painting	2.0
Sitting, writing	1.9–2.2
Playing cards	2.2
Playing piano	2.5
Playing violin	2.7
Driving car	2.8
Canoeing, 2.5 mph	3.0
Horseback riding, slow	3.0
Playing volleyball	3.5
Playing with children	3.5
Playing drums	4.0–4.2
Sculling, 51 m/min, 12 mph	4.1
Bowling	4.4
Cycling, 5.5 mph	4.5
Golf	5.0
Archery	5.2
Dancing	5.5

Gardening, weeding	5.6
Recreational swimming	6–7.0
Tennis	7.1
Trotting on a horse	8.0
Spading	8.6
Gardening, digging	8.6
Playing football	8.9
Skiing	9.9
Playing soccer	10.2
Climbing slope	10.7
Cycling, 13 mph	11.0
Swimming, breaststroke, 40 yd/min	10.0
Swimming, sidestroke, 20 yd/min	11.0
Swimming, backstroke, 40 yd/min	11.5
Swimming, crawl, 45 yd/min	11.5

Occupations

Clerical Work

Electric typewriter, 30 w/min	1.16
Electric typewriter, 40 w/min	1.31
Mechanical typewriter, 30 w/min	1.39
Mechanical typewriter, 40 w/min	1.48
Misc. office work, sitting	1.6
Misc. office work, standing	1.8

Light Engineering Work

Watch and clock repair	1.6
Light assembly line	1.8
Draftsman	1.8
Armature winding	2.2
Light machine work	2.4
Radio assembly	2.7

Printing Industry

Hand composition	2.2
Printing	2.2
Paper laying	2.5

Leather Trade

    Polishing shoes   1.8

    Filing soles   2.3

    Fixing soles   2.4

    Shoe repairing   2.7

    Shoe manufacturing   3.0

Press Goods Industry

    Pressing household utensils   3.8

Locksmith

    Filing with large file   3.3–3.7

    Five other processes   2.1–2.9

Tailor

    Hand sewing   2.0–2.9

    Cutting   2.4–2.7

    Machine sewing   2.8–2.9

    Pressing   3.5–4.3

    Ironing   4.2

Mail Carrier

    Climbing stairs   8.0

    Postal load, 24.2 lb (11 kg)   9.8

    Postal load, 35.2 lb (16 kg)   9.8–13.8

Pick, shovel, and wheelbarrow

    Shoveling, 17.6-lb (8-kg) load, 12 throws/min, 1 meter lift   7.5

    Shoveling, 17.6-lb (8-kg) load, 12 throws/min, 2 meter lift   9.5

    Shoveling, 16 lb (7 kg)   8.5

    Wheelbarrow, 115 lb (52 kg)   5.0

    Hoeing with pick   7.0

Building industry

    Measuring wood   2.4

    Machine sawing   2.4

    Light work laying stones or bricks   3.4

    Measuring and sawing   3.5

    Misc. work, carrying   3.6

    Shaping stones with mason's hammer   3.8

Making wall with bricks and mortar	4.0
Plastering	4.1
Joining floor boards	4.4
Mixing cement	4.7
Chiseling	5.7
Sawing softwood	6.3
Drilling hardwood	7.0
Sawing hardwood	6.3
Planing hardwood	9.1
Using heavy hammer	6.3–9.8

Miscellaneous

Tractor	4.2
Plowing	5.9
Haying	7.3
Mowing lawn by hand	7.3
Felling a tree	8.0
Tending a furnace	10.2
Climbing a hill or set of stairs with a 22-lb (10-kg) load, 54 ft/min	16.2

Appendix H

Resources

AMERICAN ASSOCIATION OF
DIABETES EDUCATORS
Suite 1400
500 N. Michigan Ave.
Chicago, IL 60611
1-800-338-DMED or
(312) 661-1700
*Educational material and
information about Diabetes
Educators*

THE AMERICAN DIABETES
ASSOCIATION
1660 Duke Street
Alexandria, VA 22313
1-800-232-3472
*Educational material, research
programs, and association
information*

AMERICAN DIAGNOSTICS, INC.
1301 W. 22d, Suite 312
Oakbrook, IL 60521
(708) 572-0590

AMERICAN FOUNDATION
FOR THE BLIND
15 West 16th St.
New York, NY 10011
1-800-232-5463
*Catalog, supplies, and information
for the blind*
(703) 345-6617
Product Center

AMERICAN MEDICAL SYSTEMS, INC.
1101 Bren Road, East
Minnetonka, MN 55343
*AMS Hydroflex prosthesis, AMS
600 prosthesis, AMS 700 CX
prosthesis*

C. R. BARD, INC.
Urological Division
Covington, GA 30209
*ESKA Jonas Silicon-Silver penile
prosthesis*

BECTON DICKINSON
CONSUMER PRODUCTS
One Becton Drive
Franklin Lakes, NJ 07417-1883
1-800-526-4650 or
1-800-237-4554
*Educational material and product
information, syringes*

BOEHRINGER MANNHEIM
DIAGNOSTICS, INC.
9115 Hague Rd.
P. O. Box 50100
Indianapolis, IN 46250-0100
1-800-428-5076
*Educational material and product
information, blood glucose meters*

CAN-AM CARE CORP.
Cimetra Industrial Park
Box 98
Chazy, N.Y. 12921
1-800-461-7448
*Lancets, glucose tabs, blood
glucose test strips*

CANADIAN DIABETES ASSOCIATION
78 Bond Street
Toronto, Ontario, M5B 2J8
Canada
(416) 362-4440

CHRONIMED, SUITE 250
Ridgedale Office Center
13911 Ridgedale Dr.
Minneapolis, MN 55305
1-800-944-5951

DACOMED CORPORATION
1701 East 79th Street
Minneapolis, MN 55420
DuraPhaw prosthesis, OmniPhase prosthesis, Snap-Gauge

DIABETES CENTER, INC.
Ridgedale Office Center
Suite 250
Minneapolis, MN 55394
(612) 541-0239

DIABETES SUPPLIES, INC.
8181 Stadium Dr.
Houston, TX 77054
1-800-622-5587
Supplies

DIABETES TRAVELER
P.O. Box 8223 RW
Stamford, CT 06905
Information on traveling

DISETRONIC MEDICAL SYSTEMS
13005 16th Ave. N., Suite 500
Plymonth, MN 55441
1-800-688-5698
Insulin infusion pump

DIVA MEDICAL SYSTEMS
Gainor Medical USA, Inc.
P.O. Box 931217
Long Beach, CA 90809-3129
1-800-825-8282
Lancets, Blood glucose monitoring systems

ELI LILLY AND COMPANY
CONSUMER RELATIONS
Lilly Corp. Center
Indianapolis, IN 46285
(317) 276-2000
Educational material and product information

GOLDWARD MEDICAL ID JEWELRY
P.O. Box 22335
San Diego, CA 92192
1-800-699-7311
Identification jewelry

HEALTH EDUCATION ASSOCIATES, INC.
8 Jan Sebastian Way, Unit 13
Sandwich, MA 02563
(508) 888-8044

HOME DIAGNOSTICS, INC.
6 Industrial Way West
Eatontown, NJ 07724
1-800-342-7226 (except NJ)
(201) 542-7788 (NJ only)
Blood glucose meter

ICN PHARMACEUTICALS, INC.
3300 Hyland Ave.
Costa Mesa, CA 92626
(714) 545-0100
Supplies

IDENTALERT
The Guardian Foundation
5400 Glenwood Ave., S-204
Raleigh, NC 27612
(919) 847-1600
Medical identification

INDEPENDENT LIVING AIDS, INC.
27 East Mall
Plainview, NY 11803
(516) 752-8080
Supplies

INTERNATIONAL DIABETES
FEDERATION
40 Washington Street
Brussels, Belgium 1050

JUVENILE DIABETES FOUNDATION
432 Park Avenue South
New York, NY 10016-8013
1-800-223-1138 or (212) 889-7575
*Educational material and
information*

JUVENILE DIABETES FOUNDATION
INTERNATIONAL
The Diabetes Research
Foundation
432 Park Avenue South
New York, NY 10016-8013
1-800-223-1138

LIFESCAN, INC.
1051 S. Milpitas Blvd.
Milpitas, CA 95035
1-800-227-8862
Blood glucose meter

MARKWELL MEDICAL
P.O. Box 085173
Racine, WI 53408
(414) 632-3841
Supplies

MEDIC ALERT FOUNDATION
INTERNATIONAL
Turlock, CA 95381
1-800-432-5378
Medical identification

MEDISENSE, INC.
128 Sidney Street
Cambridge, MA 02139
1-800-527-3339
(617) 492-2373
Sensors

MENTOR CORPORATION
600 Pine Avenue
Goleta, CA 93117
*Mentor GFS penile prosthesis,
Mentor penile prosthesis, Small-
Carrion prosthesis*

MILES, INC.
Diagnostic Division
P.O. Box 70
Elkhart, IN 46515
1-800-348-8100
*Educational material and product
information, blood glucose meters*

MINIMED TECHNOLOGIES, INC.
12744 San Fernando Rd.
Sylmar, CA 91342
1-800-933-3322
Insulin infusion pump

NATIONAL DIABETES INFORMATION
CLEARINGHOUSE
Box NDIC
Bethesda, MD 20892
(301) 468-2162

NATIONAL EMERGENCY MEDICINE
ASSOCIATION (NEMA)
306 West Joppa Road
Towson, MD 21204
1-800-332-6362 (except MD)
(301) 494-0300 (MD only)
*Daytime hours and recorded
answering device; information*

NOVO-NORDISK
PHARMACEUTICALS, INC.
100 Overlook Center
Suite 200
Princeton, NJ 08540
(609) 987-5800
1-800-223-0872
*Educational material and product
information, Insulins*

ORANGE MEDICAL INSTRUMENTS
23142 Alcalde, Unit C
Laguna Hills, CA 92653
1-800-527-1151 (except CA)
1-800-345-2993 (CA only)
Blood glucose meter

OSBON MEDICAL SYSTEMS
1246 Jones Street
P.O. Drawer 1478
Augusta, GA 30903-9990
ErecAid System

RESOURCES FOR REHABILITATION
33 Bedford Street, Suite 19A
Lexington, MA 02173
(617) 862-6455

THE REVIVE SYSTEM CORPORATION
156 Broad Street, Box 592
Lake Geneva, WI 53147
Revive System

SHERWOOD MEDICAL
1831 Olive St.
St. Louis, MO 63103
1-800-367-5036 or (314) 241-5700
Supplies

SMITH-COLLINS
PHARMACEUTICAL, INC.
889 South Matlack Street
West Chester, PA 19382
(215) 251-7400
Response System

SUGAR-FREE CENTER
5623 Matilize Ave.
Van Nuys, CA 91401
(818) 994-1093
Newsletter, catalog, supplies, and information

SURGITEK
Medical Engineering
Corporation
3037 Mt. Pleasant Street
Racine, WI 53404
(414) 639-7205
Flexi-Flate prosthesis, Flexi-rod prosthesis, Uni-Flate 1000

SYNERGIST LIMITED
6910 Fannin, Suite 100
Houston, TX 77030
(713) 796-9191
Synergist Erection System

TERUMO CORPORATION
Consumer Products Division
2100 Cottontail La.
Somerset, NJ 08873
1-800-252-6782
Syringes

ULSTER SCIENTIFIC
P.O. Box 902
Highland, NY 12528
1-800-431-8233 (except NY)
1-800-522-2257 (NY only)
Product information

UNIVERSITY OF MICHIGAN
Media Library
R4440 Kresge III, Box 0518
Ann Arbor, MI 48109-0518
(313) 763-2074

UPJOHN COMPANY
7000 Portage Road
Kalamazoo, MI 49001
(616) 323-4000
Oral agents

VITAJET PRECISION
INSTRUMENTS, INC.
Mada Equipment Co., Inc.
600 Commerce Rd.
Carlstadt, NJ 07072
1-800-848-2538
Jet injectors

Appendix I

Diabetes Associations by State

ALABAMA

AMERICAN DIABETES ASSOCIATION
ALABAMA AFFILIATE, INC.
3 Office Park Circle, Suite 115
Birmingham, AL 35223
1-800-824-7891, (205) 870-5172,
or *(205) 870-5173*

ALASKA

AMERICAN DIABETES ASSOCIATION
ALASKA AFFILIATE, INC.
1301 Penland Parkway,
Suite G-34
Anchorage, AK 99508
(907) 279-6015

ARIZONA

AMERICAN DIABETES ASSOCIATION
ARIZONA AFFILIATE, INC.
2328 W. Royal Palm Rd., Suite D
Phoenix, AZ 85021
(602) 995-0004

ARKANSAS

AMERICAN DIABETES ASSOCIATION
ARKANSAS AFFILIATE, INC.
11500 N. Rodney Parham
Executive Suite Bldg.
Suite 19 & 20
Little Rock, AR 72212
(501) 221-7444

CALIFORNIA

AMERICAN DIABETES ASSOCIATION
CALIFORNIA AFFILIATE, INC.
10445 Old Placerville Rd.
Sacramento, CA 95827
(916) 369-0999

COLORADO

AMERICAN DIABETES ASSOCIATION
COLORADO AFFILIATE, INC.
2450 S. Downing Street
Denver, CO 80210
(303) 778-7556

CONNECTICUT

AMERICAN DIABETES ASSOCIATION
CONNECTICUT AFFILIATE, INC.
300 Research Parkway
Meriden, CT 06450
(203) 639-038

DELAWARE

AMERICAN DIABETES ASSOCIATION
DELAWARE AFFILIATE, INC.
2713 Lancaster Avenue
Wilmington, DE 19805
(302) 656-0030

DISTRICT OF COLUMBIA

AMERICAN DIABETES ASSOCIATION
WASHINGTON, D.C. AREA
AFFILIATE, INC.
1211 Connecticut Avenue, N.W.,
Suite 501
Washington, D.C. 20036
(202) 331-8303

FLORIDA

AMERICAN DIABETES ASSOCIATION
FLORIDA AFFILIATE, INC.
1101 N. Lake Destiny Rd.,
Suite 415
Maitland, FL 32751
1-800-741-5698 or *(407) 660-9926*

GEORGIA

AMERICAN DIABETES ASSOCIATION
GEORGIA AFFILIATE, INC.
3783 Presidential Parkway,
Suite 102
Atlanta, GA 30340
(404) 454-8401

HAWAII

AMERICAN DIABETES ASSOCIATION
HAWAII AFFILIATE, INC.
810 N. Vineyard Blvd., Suite 11
Honolulu, HI 96817
(808) 814-3997

IDAHO

AMERICAN DIABETES ASSOCIATION
IDAHO AFFILIATE, INC.
1528 Vista
Boise, ID 83705
(208) 342-2774

ILLINOIS

AMERICAN DIABETES ASSOCIATION
DOWNSTATE ILLINOIS AFFILIATE, INC.
2580 Federal Drive
Decatur, IL 62526
(217) 875-9011

AMERICAN DIABETES ASSOCIATION
NORTHERN ILLINOIS AFFILIATE, INC.
6 N. Michigan Avenue, Suite 1202
Chicago, IL 60602
(312) 346-1805

INDIANA

AMERICAN DIABETES ASSOCIATION
INDIANA AFFILIATE, INC.
222 S. Downey Avenue, Suite 320
Indianapolis, IN 46219
(317) 352-9226

IOWA

AMERICAN DIABETES ASSOCIATION
IOWA AFFILIATE, INC.
6656 Douglas Ave.
Des Moines, IA 50322
1-800-678-4232 or *(515) 276-2237*

KANSAS

AMERICAN DIABETES ASSOCIATION
KANSAS AFFILIATE, INC.
3210 E. Douglas
Wichita, KS 67208
(316) 684-6091

KENTUCKY

AMERICAN DIABETES ASSOCIATION
KENTUCKY AFFILIATE, INC.
745 West Main, Suite 150
Louisville, KY 40202
(502) 589-3837

LOUISIANA

AMERICAN DIABETES ASSOCIATION
LOUISIANA AFFILIATE, INC.
9420 Lindale Avenue, Suite B
Baton Rouge, LA 70815
(504) 927-7732

MAINE

AMERICAN DIABETES ASSOCIATION
MAINE AFFILIATE, INC.
P.O. Box 2208 (mailing address)
8 Crosby Street (building
address)
Augusta, ME 04388
(207) 623-2232

MARYLAND

AMERICAN DIABETES ASSOCIATION
MARYLAND AFFILIATE, INC.
2 Reservoir Circle, Suite 203
Baltimore, MD 21208
(301) 486-5516

MASSACHUSETTS

AMERICAN DIABETES ASSOCIATION
MASSACHUSETTS AFFILIATE, INC.
P.O. Box 122 (mailing address)
400 Speen Street (building
address)
Framingham, MA 01701
(508) 879-1776

MICHIGAN

AMERICAN DIABETES ASSOCIATION
MICHIGAN AFFILIATE, INC.
The Clausen Building North Unit
23100 Providence Drive,
Suite 400
Southfield, MI 48075
(313) 552-0480

MINNESOTA

AMERICAN DIABETES ASSOCIATION
MINNESOTA AFFILIATE, INC.
715 Florida West Building,
Suite 307
Golden Valley, MN 55426
(612) 920-6796

MISSISSIPPI

AMERICAN DIABETES ASSOCIATION
MISSISSIPPI AFFILIATE, INC.
16 Northtown Drive, Suite 100
Jackson, MS 39211
(601) 957-7878

MISSOURI

AMERICAN DIABETES ASSOCIATION
MISSOURI AFFILIATE, INC.
P.O. Box 1674 (mailing address)
213 Adams Street, Suite 201
(building address)
Jefferson City, MO 65102
(314) 636-5552

MONTANA

AMERICAN DIABETES ASSOCIATION
MONTANA AFFILIATE, INC.
Box 2411 (mailing address)
Great Falls, MT 59403
600 Central Plaza, Suite 201
(building address)
Great Falls, MT 59403
(406) 761-0908

NEBRASKA

AMERICAN DIABETES ASSOCIATION
NEBRASKA AFFILIATE, INC.
12828 Augusta Avenue
Omaha, NE 68144
(402) 333-5556

NEVADA
AMERICAN DIABETES ASSOCIATION
NEVADA AFFILIATE, INC.
4045 S. Spencer, Suite A-62
Las Vegas, NV 89119
(702) 369-9995

NEW HAMPSHIRE
AMERICAN DIABETES ASSOCIATION
NEW HAMPSHIRE AFFILIATE, INC.
(603) 627-9579

NEW JERSEY
AMERICAN DIABETES ASSOCIATION
NEW JERSEY AFFILIATE, INC.
P.O. Box 6423 (mailing address)
312 N. Adamsville Road
(street address)
Bridgewater, NJ 08807
(201) 725-7878

NEW MEXICO
AMERICAN DIABETES ASSOCIATION
NEW MEXICO AFFILIATE, INC.
525 San Pedro, N.E., Suite 101
Albuquerque, NM 87108
(505) 266-5716

NEW YORK
AMERICAN DIABETES ASSOCIATION
NEW YORK DOWNSTATE
AFFILIATE, INC.
149 Madison Avenue, 7th floor
New York, NY 10016
(212) 725-4925

AMERICAN DIABETES ASSOCIATION
NEW YORK UPSTATE AFFILIATE, INC.
523 W. Manlius Street
East Syracuse, NY 13050
(315) 463-9111

NORTH CAROLINA
AMERICAN DIABETES ASSOCIATION
NORTH CAROLINA AFFILIATE, INC.
2315-A Sunset Avenue
Rocky Mount, NC 27801
(919) 937-4121

NORTH DAKOTA
AMERICAN DIABETES ASSOCIATION
NORTH DAKOTA AFFILIATE, INC.
P.O. Box 234 (mailing address)
Grand Forks, ND 58206-0234
101 N. 3rd Street, Suite 502
(street address)
Grand Forks, ND 58201
(701) 746-4427

OHIO
AMERICAN DIABETES ASSOCIATION
OHIO AFFILIATE, INC.
937 North High Street
Columbus, OH 43085
(614) 436-1917

OKLAHOMA
AMERICAN DIABETES ASSOCIATION
OKLAHOMA AFFILIATE, INC.
Warren Professional Building
6465 S. Yale Avenue, Suite 519
Tulsa, OK 74136
1-800-722-5448 or *(918) 492-3839*

OREGON

AMERICAN DIABETES ASSOCIATION
OREGON AFFILIATE, INC.
3607 S.W. Corbett Street
Portland, OR 97201
(503) 228-0849

PENNSYLVANIA

AMERICAN DIABETES ASSOCIATION
PENNSYLVANIA AFFILIATE, INC.
5020 Ritter Rd., Suite 103
Mechanicsburg, PA 17055
(717) 691-6170; (800) 357-5800

PUERTO RICO

AMERICAN DIABETES ASSOCIATION
PUERTO RICO AFFILIATE, INC.
Avenue Jesus T. Pineiro
(Central) 1161 Altos
Puerto Nuevo, PR 00920
(809) 793-1276

RHODE ISLAND

AMERICAN DIABETES ASSOCIATION
RHODE ISLAND AFFILIATE, INC.
Warwick Executive Park
250 Centerville Road
Warwick, RI 02886
(401) 738-5570

SOUTH CAROLINA

AMERICAN DIABETES ASSOCIATION
SOUTH CAROLINA AFFILIATE, INC.
P.O. Box 50782 (mailing address)
2711 Middlebury Drive,
Suite 311
(building address)
Columbia, SC 29250
(803) 799-4246

SOUTH DAKOTA

AMERICAN DIABETES ASSOCIATION
SOUTH DAKOTA AFFILIATE, INC.
P.O. Box 659 (mailing address)
Sioux Falls, SD 57101
1100 E. Euclid Avenue
(building address)
(605) 335-7670

TENNESSEE

AMERICAN DIABETES ASSOCIATION
TENNESSEE AFFILIATE, INC.
Green Hills Court
4205 Hillsboro Rd., Suite 200
Nashville, TN 37215
(615) 298-9919

TEXAS

AMERICAN DIABETES ASSOCIATION
TEXAS AFFILIATE, INC.
8140 N. Mopac, Bldg. 1, Suite 130
Austin, TX 78759
(512) 343-6981

UTAH

AMERICAN DIABETES ASSOCIATION
UTAH AFFILIATE, INC.
643 East 400 South
Salt Lake City, UT 84102
(801) 363-3024

VERMONT

AMERICAN DIABETES ASSOCIATION
VERMONT AFFILIATE, INC.
431 Pine Street
Maltex Building
Burlington, VT 05401
(802) 862-3882

VIRGINIA

AMERICAN DIABETES ASSOCIATION
VIRGINIA AFFILIATE, INC.
404 8th Street, N.E., Suite C
Charlottesville, VA 22901
(804) 293-4953

WASHINGTON

AMERICAN DIABETES ASSOCIATION
WASHINGTON AFFILIATE, INC.
557 Roy Street
Seattle, WA 98109
(206) 282-4616

WEST VIRGINIA

AMERICAN DIABETES ASSOCIATION
WEST VIRGINIA AFFILIATE, INC.
5626 MacCorkle
Kanawha City, WV 25364
1-800-232-6366 or *(304) 925-6685*

WISCONSIN

AMERICAN DIABETES ASSOCIATION
WISCONSIN AFFILIATE, INC.
2949 N. Mayfair Road, Suite 306
Wauwatosa, WE 53222
(414) 778-5500

WYOMING

AMERICAN DIABETES ASSOCIATION
WYOMING AFFILIATE, INC.
2526 6th Avenue North
Billings, MT 59101
(406) 256-0616 or *(800) 877-0106*

Appendix J

Camps for Children with Diabetes

ARIZONA

CAMP AZDA
2328 W. Royal Palm Rd., Suite D
Phoenix, AZ 85021

Contact:
Executive Director
American Diabetes Association
Arizona Affiliate, Inc.
7337 North 19th Avenue
P.O. Box 37579
Phoenix, AZ 85069
(602) 995-1515

Sponsored by:
American Diabetes Association
Arizona Affiliate, Inc.

Ages 7–12½, thirteen-day session

CALIFORNIA

BEARSKIN MEADOW CAMP
Kings Canyon National Park, CA

Contact:
Ronald Brown
1954 Mt. Diablo Blvd., Suite A
Walnut Creek, CA 94596
(510) 937-3393

Sponsored by:
Diabetic Youth Foundation

Ages 6–18, two-week session
Family camps, three-day session

CAMP CHINNOCK
Angelus Oaks, CA

Contact:
Joanie Johnston
10445 Old Placerville Rd.
Sacramento, CA 95827
(916) 369-0999

Sponsored by:
ADA California Affiliate

Ages 7–9, eleven-day session
Ages 10–13, eleven-day session
Ages 10–14, eleven-day session
Ages 14–16, eleven-day session

CAMP DE LOS NIÑOS
Boulder Creek
Santa Cruz Mountains, CA

Contact:
Madelyn Zelman
1261 Lincoln Ave., Suite 208
San Jose, CA 95125
(408) 287-3785

Sponsored by:
Santa Clara Valley Diabetes
Society

Ages 6–12, one-week session
Ages 13–16, one-week session,
with optional backpack trip in an
extended session

COLORADO

CHILDREN'S DIABETES CAMP
Contact:
Browning Lummis
2450 S. Downing
Denver, CO 80210(303) 778-7556
Sponsored by:
ADA Colorado Affiliate
Ages 8–17, six-day session

CONNECTICUT

YOUTH SUMMER CAMP PROGRAM
Contact:
Liana Desroches
300 Research Parkway
Meriden, CT 06450
(203) 639-0385
Sponsored by:
ADA Connecticut Affiliate

DISTRICT OF COLUMBIA

See Maryland listing

FLORIDA

FLORIDA CAMP FOR CHILDREN AND
YOUTH
Contact:
Rosalee Bandyopadhyay
P.O. Box 141356, University
Station
Gainesville, FL 32604
(904) 392-4123

GEORGIA

CAMP LIWIDIA
Contact:
Todd Garrett
3783 Presidential Pkwy.,
Suite 102
Atlanta, GA 30340
(404) 454-8401
Sponsored by:
ADA Georgia Affiliate

ILLINOIS

See also listings under Wisconsin
and Michigan

CAMP GRANADA
RR 5
Jacksonville, IL 62650
Contact:
Donna Scott
2580 Federal Drive
Decatur, IL 62526
(217) 875-9011
Sponsored by:
ADA Downstate Illinois Affiliate
Ages 8–15, six-day session

YMCA CAMP DUNCAN
Contact:
Suzanne Apsey
6 North Michigan Avenue,
Suite 1202
Chicago, IL 60602
(312) 352-9226
Sponsored by:
ADA Northern Illinois Affiliate

INDIANA

CAMP JOHN WARVEL

Contact:
Director of Programs
222 S. Downey Avenue, Suite 320
Indianapolis, IN 46219
(317) 352-9226
Sponsored by:
American Diabetes Association
Indiana Affiliate, Inc.
Ages 7–15, six- and fourteen-day sessions
Ages 14–18, fourteen-day session

IOWA

CAMP HERTKO HOLLOW
Contact:
Beth Volz
6656 Douglas Avenue
Des Moines, IA 50322
(515) 276-2237
Sponsored by:
ADA Iowa Affiliate
Ages 8–16, six-day session

KANSAS

CAMP DISCOVERY
Contact:
Camp Coordinator
American Diabetes Association
Kansas Affiliate, Inc.
3210 E. Douglas
Wichita, KS 67208
(316) 684-6091
Sponsored by:
American Diabetes Association
Kansas Affiliate, Inc.
Ages 8–10, four-day session
Ages 11–13, six-day session
Ages 14–17, six-day session

LOUISIANA

LOUISIANA LIONS LEAGUE CAMP
Contact:
Area Director
American Diabetes Association
Louisiana Affiliate, Inc.
9420 Lindale Avenue, Suite B
Baton Rouge, LA 70815
(504) 927-7732
Sponsored by:
American Diabetes Association
Louisiana Affiliate, Inc.
Ages 6–10, six-day session

MAINE

CAMP KEE-TO-KIN
Contact:
Joan Maccraken, M.D.
489 State Street
Bangor, ME 04401-6674
Sponsored by:
Eastern Maine Medical Center

CAMP GLYNDON
Contact:
Camp Director
2 Reservoir Circle, Suite 203
Baltimore, MD 21208
(410) 486-5515
Sponsored by:
DAD Maryland Affiliate

MARYLAND

CAMP GLYNDON
407 Central Avenue
Reisterstown, MD 21136
Contact:
Camp Director
3701 Old Court Road, #20
Baltimore, MD 21208
(301) 486-5515

Sponsored by:
American Diabetes Association
Maryland Affiliate, Inc.

Ages 7–9, five-day session
Ages 10–13, twelve-day session
Ages 13–15, twelve-day session
Family, five-day session

MASSACHUSETTS

CLARA BARTON CAMP FOR GIRLS WITH DIABETES, INC.

Contact:
Administrator
Clara Barton Camp
P.O. Box 356
North Oxford, MA 01537
(508) 987-2056

Sponsored by:
Clara Barton Camp for Girls
with Diabetes, Inc.
American Diabetes Association
Massachusetts Affiliate, Inc.

Ages 6–17, twelve-day session

ELLIOTT P. JOSLIN CAMP FOR BOYS WITH DIABETES

Richardson Corner Road
P.O. Box 100
Charlton, MA 01507

Contact:
Camp Administration
Camp Joslin
1 Joslin Place
Boston, MA 02215
(617) 732-2455

Sponsored by:
Joslin Diabetes Center
American Diabetes Association
Massachusetts Affiliate, Inc.

Ages 7–16¹/₂, twelve- and
nineteen-day sessions
Ages 12–16¹/₂, five-day session

MICHIGAN

CAMP MIDICHA

4205 Hollenbeck Road
Columbiaville, MI 48421

Contact:
Director of Youth Services
American Diabetes Association
23100 Providence Drive,
Suite 400
Southfield, MI 48075
(313) 552-0480

Sponsored by:
American Diabetes Association
Michigan Affiliate, Inc.

Ages 6–10, six-day session
Ages 8–12, six-day session
Ages 10–14, thirteen-day session
Ages 12–16, thirteen-day session

CAMP MIDICHA, U.P.

Bay Cliff Health Camp
Big Bay, MI 49808

Contact:
Director of Youth Services
23100 Providence Drive
Suite 400
Southfield, MI 48075
(313) 552-0480

Sponsored by:
American Diabetes Association
Michigan Affiliate, Inc.

Ages 8–16, nine-day session

TEEN ADVENTURE CAMP

Contact:
Mary Delacey
6 North Michigan Avenue,
Suite 1202
Chicago, IL 60602
(312) 346-1805

Sponsored by:
ADA Northern Illinois Affiliate

MINNESOTA

See Wisconsin listing for camp sponsored by Minnesota Affiliate

MISSISSIPPI

TWIN LAKES CAMP

Contact:
Mary Forturne
16 Northtown Drive, S-100
Jackson, MS 39211
(601) 957-7878

Sponsored by:
ADA Mississippi Affiliate

Ages 7–11, six-day session
Ages 12–16, six-day session

MISSOURI

CAMP EDI
YMCA Trout Lodge
RR 2
Potosi, MO 63664

Contact:
Camp Director
1316 Parkade Blvd.
P.O. Box 1013
Columbia, MO 65205
(314) 443-8611

Sponsored by:
American Diabetes Association
Missouri Affiliate, Inc.

Ages 7–15, twelve-day session

CAMP HICKORY HILL
P.O. Box 1942
Columbia, MO 65205

Contact:
Medical Director
113 West Broadway
Columbia, MO 65203
(314) 443-2447

Sponsored by:
American Diabetes Association
Missouri Affiliate, Inc.

Ages 8–12, ten-day session
Ages 13–17, twelve-day session

CAMP RED-BIRD

Contact:
Stephanie Tranen, MPH, RD
9440 Manchester Rd., Suite 104
St. Louis, MO 63199
(314) 968-3196

Sponsored by:
American Diabetes Association

CAMP SHAWNEE
Camp Fire, Inc.
P.O. Box 22
Waldron, MO 64092

Contact:
Camp Director
1316 Parkade Blvd.
P.O. Box 1013
Columbia, MO 65205
(314) 443-8611

Sponsored by:
American Diabetes Association
Missouri Affiliate, Inc.

Ages 7–14, six-day session

MONTANA

CAMP DIAMONT

Contact:
Executive Director
American Diabetes Association
Montana Affiliate, Inc.
Box 2411
Great Falls, MT 59403
(406) 761-0908

Sponsored by:
American Diabetes Association
Montana Affiliate, Inc.

Ages 8–14, six-day session

NEW HAMPSHIRE

CAMP CAREFREE

Contact:
American Diabetes Association
New Hampshire Affiliate, Inc.
Box 595
Manchester, NH 03105
(603) 627-9579

Sponsored by:
American Diabetes Association
New Hampshire Affiliate, Inc.

Ages 8–15, twelve-day session

NEW JERSEY

CAMP NEJEDA

Contact:
Camp Director
Saddleback Road
P.O. Box 156
Stillwater, NJ 07875
(201) 383-2611

Sponsored by:
Camp Nejeda Foundation, Inc.
American Diabetes Association
New Jersey Affiliate, Inc.

Ages 5–11, six-day session
Ages 7–11, thirteen-day session
Ages 12–15, thirteen-day sessions
Age 16, Counselor-in-Training
(CIT) Program, twenty-four-day
session

NEW YORK

CAMP SUNSHINE
Rotary Sunshine Camp
809 Five Points Road
Rush, NY 14543

Contact:
Program Director
American Diabetes Association
Rochester Regional Chapter
1650 Elmwood Avenue
Rochester, NY 14620
(716) 271-1260

Sponsored by:
American Diabetes Association
New York Upstate Affiliate, Inc.

Ages 8–16, nine-day session

NORTH CAROLINA

CAMP HANES
Route 5, Box 99
King, NC 27021

Contact:
Executive Director
North Carolina Affiliate, Inc.
2315-A Sunset Avenue
Rocky Mount, NC 27804
1-800-682-9692 or *(919) 937-4121*

Sponsored by:
American Diabetes Association
North Carolina Affiliate, Inc.

Ages 8–15, six-day session

NORTH DAKOTA

CAMP SIOUX
Turtle River State Park
Arvilla, ND 58214

Contact:
Executive Director
American Diabetes Association
North Dakota Affiliate, Inc.
P.O. Box 234
Grand Forks, ND 58201
(701) 746-4427

Sponsored by:
American Diabetes Association
North Dakota Affiliate, Inc.

Ages 8–14, six-day session

OHIO

CAMP KORELITZ
Contact:
Kevin Vance
3605 Pape Avenue
Cincinnati, OH 45208
(513) 281-0002

OKLAHOMA

CAMP NE OCA DA
Contact:
Phyllis Raines
7230 E. 64th Place
Tulsa, OK 74133
(918) 492-5828

Sponsored by:
American Diabetes Association

CAMP O'LEARY/KNO-KETO
YMCA Camp Classen
Route 1
Davis, OK 73030

Contact:
Program Coordinator
American Diabetes Association
Oklahoma Affiliate, Inc.
3909 Classen Blvd., Suite 101
Oklahoma City, OK 73118
(405) 525-0222

Sponsored by:
American Diabetes Association
Oklahoma Affiliate, Inc.

Ages 8–16, TBA

CAMP RED-BUD
Contact:
Denny Krick, Ed.D.
2501 Mercer Drive
Enid, OK 73701
(405) 233-0650

Sponsored by:
Garfield County Health
Department

OREGON

GALES CREEK CAMP
HCR 71, Box 1205
Forest Grove, OR 97116

Contact:
American Diabetes Association
Oregon Affiliate, Inc.
6915 SW Macadam, #130
Portland, OR 97219
(503) 245-2010

Sponsored by:
American Diabetes Association
Oregon Affiliate, Inc.

Grades 1–3, six-day session
Grades 4–6, thirteen-day session
Grades 7–8, thirteen-day session
Grades 9–11, thirteen-day session

PENNSYLVANIA

CAMP CRESTFIELD

Contact:
Camp Director
Camp Crestfield
RD 2, Box 71
Slippery Rock, PA 16057
(412) 794-4022

Sponsored by:
American Diabetes Association
Western Pennsylvania
Affiliate, Inc.

Grades 2–5, six-day session
Grades 6–10, six-day session

CAMP FIREFLY
Haim Road
Spring Mount, PA 19478

Contact:
Youth Services Director
American Diabetes Association
Greater Philadelphia
Affiliate, Inc.
21 South Fifth Street, Suite 570
Philadelphia, PA 19106
(215) 627-7718

Sponsored by:
American Diabetes Association
Greater Philadelphia
Affiliate, Inc.

Ages 6–10 (girls), thirteen-day
session
Ages 6–10 (boys), thirteen-day
session
Ages 11–15 (girls), thirteen-day
session
Ages 11–15 (boys), thirteen-day
session

CAMP SETEBAID
RD 3
Shickshinny, PA 18655

Contact:
Michelle Knight
5020 Ritter Road, Suite 106
Mechanicsburg, PA 17055
(717) 691-6170

Sponsored by:
ADA Pennsylvania Affiliate

Ages 8–12, six-day session

DR. BARCLAY'S CAMP FOR
DIABETIC CHILDREN
c/o ECDA
1741 West 26th Street
Erie, PA 16508
(814) 922-3219

Sponsored by:
Erie County Diabetes Association
American Diabetes Association
Western Pennsylvania
Affiliate, Inc.

Ages 8–15, seven- and fourteen-
day sessions

SOUTH CAROLINA

CAMP ADAM FISHER
Contact:
Chairman, Youth Services
American Diabetes Association
South Carolina Affiliate, Inc.
2200 Green Pines Road
Columbia, SC 29206
(803) 736-0329

Sponsored by:
American Diabetes Association
South Carolina Affiliate, Inc.

Ages 7–18, nine-day session

SOUTH DAKOTA

CAMP HAUNZ
Contact:
Joyce Kaatz, RN
1100 S. Euclid
Sioux Falls, SD 57117-5039
(605) 333-1000 Beeper 1392

TENNESSEE

CAMP WACK-A-DOO
Contact:
Stephanie Hasenwalder
317 Oak Street, #103
Chattanooga, TN 37403
(615) 756-8709
Sponsored by:
American Diabetes Association

CAMP RISING SUN
Contact:
Ben Harrington
8906 Kingston Pike, 105C
Knoxville, TN 37023
(615) 531-1129
Sponsored by:
American Diabetes Association

CAMP SUGAR FALLS
Contact:
Kristin Robbins
4205 Hillsboro Rd., Suite 200
Nashville, TN 37215
(615) 298-3066
Sponsored by:
American Diabetes Association

TEXAS

CAMP SWEENEY
101 South Culberson
Gainesville, TX 76240

Contact:
P.O. Box 918
Gainesville, TX 76240
Sponsored by:
American Diabetes Association
Texas Affiliate, Inc.

Ages 6–18, nineteen-day session

TEXAS LIONS CAMP
Contact:
Texas Lions Camp
P.O. Box 247
Kerrville, TX 78029-0247
Sponsored by:
American Diabetes Association
Texas Affiliate, Inc.

Ages 7–12, nine-day session
Ages 13–17, six-day session

UTAH

CAMP DUDLEY
Contact:
Myrl Weaver
P.O. Box 2885
Yakima, WA 98907
(509) 245-1202
Sponsored by:
Yakima Family YMCA

CAMP UTADA
Contact:
Executive Director
American Diabetes Association
Utah Affiliate, Inc.
643 E. 400 South
Salt Lake City, UT 84102
(801) 363-3024
Sponsored by:
American Diabetes Association
Utah Affiliate, Inc.

Grades 2–4, six-day session
Grades 5–7, six-day session
Grades 8–11, six-day session
Family, two-day session

VIRGINIA

CAMP HOLIDAY TRAILS

Contact:
P.O. Box 5806
Charlottesville, VA 22905
(804) 977-3781

Sponsored by:
American Diabetes Association
Virginia Affiliate, Inc.

Ages 7–17, twelve-day session

CAMP JORDAN
Camp Makemie Woods
Box 39
Barhamsville, VA 23011

Contact:
Medical Director
Box 65, Medical College
of Virginia
Richmond, VA 23298
(804) 786-4094

Sponsored by:
American Diabetes Association
Virginia Affiliate, Inc.

Ages 9–15, thirteen-day session

WASHINGTON

CAMP ORKILA
YMCA Camp Orkila
P.O. Box 1149
Eastsound, WA 98245

Contact:
Program Director
American Diabetes Association
Washington Affiliate, Inc.
3201 Fremont Avenue North
Seattle, WA 98103
(206) 632-4576

Sponsored by:
American Diabetes Association
Washington Affiliate, Inc.

Grades 3–8, eleven-day session

CAMP SEALTH
Camp Fire
Route 4, Box 509
Vashon Island, WA 98070

Contact:
Dave Kamenz
8511 15th Avenue, N.E.
Seattle, WA 98115
(206) 382-5009

Sponsored by:
Camp Fire

Grades 3–12, four 8-day sessions

WISCONSIN

CAMP NEEDLEPOINT/DAYPOINT
YMCA Camp St. Croix
County Road F
Hudson, WI 54016

Contact:
Camp Director
American Diabetes Association
Minnesota Affiliate, Inc.
3005 Ottawa Avenue, South
Minneapolis, MN 55416
(612) 920-6796

Sponsored by:
American Diabetes Association
Minnesota Affiliate, Inc.

Ages 6–9, four-day session
Ages 8–16, six- and seven-day
sessions

TRIANGLE D CAMP FOR CHILDREN
WITH DIABETES
Covenant Harbor Camp
1724 Main Street
Lake Geneva, WI 53147

Contact:
Program Director
American Diabetes Association
Northern Illinois Affiliate, Inc.
6 North Michigan Avenue,
Suite 1202
Chicago, IL 60602
(312) 346-1805 or *1-800-433-4966*
(in Illinois)
Sponsored by:
American Diabetes Association
Northern Illinois Affiliate, Inc.

Ages 8–10, six-day session
Ages 11–13, six-day session

ADA/WA CAMP
2155 Lakeshore Drive
Chilton, WI 53014

Contact:
Program Director
American Diabetes Association
Wisconsin Affiliate, Inc.
10721 W. Capitol Drive
Milwaukee, WI 53222
(414) 464-9395
Sponsored by:
American Diabetes Association
Wisconsin Affiliate, Inc.

Ages 8–11, six-day session
Ages 10–17, thirteen-day session

WYOMING

CAMP HOPE
Contact:
Steve and Nancy Johnson
2710 Navarre
Casper, WY 82604
(307) 265-5865

Appendix K

Glossary of Diabetes-Related Terms

AADE American Association of Diabetes Educators. A national voluntary organization of professionals interested in education of the person and/or family with diabetes.

acetoacetic acid An acid that also contains a ketone group in its molecule.

acetone A ketone formed in greater abundance in the liver from fatty acids when glucose is not available to the cells for energy. Acetone, one of three ketones, is found in the blood and urine of people with uncontrolled diabetes and causes the breath to have a fruity odor.

acidosis An acid condition of the body resulting from abnormal amounts of acid, such as acetoacetic and beta hydroxybutyric acids. Acidosis occurs in people who are not producing insulin or who do not receive enough insulin.

ADA American Diabetes Association, Incorporated, is a national voluntary health organization of professional and lay people interested in research, service, and education in the field of diabetes.

adrenal glands Two tent-shaped organs that secrete epinephrine (see *epinephrine*) and glucocorticoids (see *glucocorticoids*) and aldosterone.

adult diabetes Now called Type II or non–insulin-dependent diabetes mellitus. See *Type II diabetes*.

alpha cells Cells that produce glucagon; found in the islets of Langerhans of the pancreas.

angiopathy Blood-vessel disease (see *microangiopathy* and *macroangiopathy*).

atrophy The shrinking of a body part due to lack of nutrition. In diabetes, this may mean a decrease in the amount of fat under the skin. This sometimes occurs at the sites of insulin injection and results in hollowed-out areas that are cosmetically undesirable.

basement membrane Layers of concentric circles, or chains, of glycoproteins separated by infrequent glucose and galactose molecules, protectively surrounding cells of the capillaries of kidney, muscle, retina of the eye, etc.

beta cells   Cells that produce insulin; found in the islet of Langerhans of the pancreas.

beta hydroxybutyric acid   One product of metabolized fat.

biguanides   Drugs, such as phenformin (DBI and DBI-TD), have also been used in treating diabetes. They do not stimulate the pancreas to produce more insulin but prevent glucose uptake from the intestine, prevent gluconeogenesis, and promote the breakdown of glucose, among other actions. Although these drugs are not now available in the U.S., a new phenformin called metformin is being tested. It is found to be less of a cause of lactic acidosis, a side effect seen in the use of the earlier drugs.

blood-glucose level   The concentration of glucose in the blood. It is commonly called blood sugar and is usually measured in milligrams per deciliter (mg/dl) or in millimoles (mMol).

brittle diabetes   A type of Type I diabetes in which the blood-glucose level fluctuates widely from high to low. Brittle diabetes can be caused by the complete loss of ability to produce any insulin, by too high an insulin dose, or by other factors. It can often be improved through a good treatment program. Also called unstable diabetes.

caesarean section   An operation in which an infant is delivered by being removed from the mother's womb through an incision in the abdomen. Infants of diabetic mothers (IDM) are frequently delivered before term by this means.

callus   A thickening of the skin caused by friction or pressure.

calorie   A unit for the measurement of heat. The heat-producing, or energy-producing, value of foods is measured in calories. A true calorie is such a small unit that 1,000 calories—a kilocalorie—is usually referred to as a calorie when discussing calorie values of food.

calorie content   The amount of heat released on the burning of one gram of food, most correctly called a kilocalorie (k).

carbohydrate   One of the three main constituents of foods. Carbohydrates are composed mainly of sugars and starches.

cardiovascular disease   Disease of the heart and large blood vessels; tends to occur more often and at a younger age in people with diabetes and may be related to how well the diabetes is controlled.

cell membrane   The material that surrounds all cells and acts to retain helpful substances, exclude harmful substances, and allow glucose to pass into the cells (with the help of insulin).

Charcot's joint Chronic progressive degeneration of the stress-bearing action of a joint (i.e. ankles).

cholesterol A mixture of lipoproteins found in blood, consisting of HDL (high-density lipoproteins), LDL (low-density lipoproteins), and VLDL (very-low-density lipoproteins). Present recommendations are to keep cholesterol levels below 200 mg/dl.

closed-loop system A self-controlled blood-glucose control system (artificial pancreas or artificial beta cell).

conventional control One or two doses of insulin with blood sugars higher than normal 50% or more of the time.

corns Hard, thickened areas of the skin caused by friction or pressure. These usually occur on the feet and may result in foot ulcers in people who have a loss of pain sensation in their feet.

DCCT Diabetes Control and Complications Trial—a 6–9 year research study involving people with Type I diabetes. The outcome with the use of intensive control can prevent or delay complications related to hyperglycemia.

dawn phenomenon An early-morning rise in blood-glucose levels, believed to be due to a delayed response in growth-hormone release.

diabetes mellitus A disease in which the body is unable to use and store glucose normally because of a decrease or lack of insulin production. Diabetes mellitus is usually inherited, but it may be caused by any process that destroys the pancreas (usually the beta cells) or alters the effectiveness of the receptor site on the cell membrane.

diabetic coma Unconsciousness occurring during ketoacidosis. Associated symptoms include dry skin and mouth, fruity odor of the breath, very deep and rapid respirations, rapid pulse, and low blood pressure. Diabetic coma is caused by a deficiency of insulin.

diabetic ketoacidosis (DKA) The most severe state of diabetes, in which there are markedly elevated glucose levels in blood and urine, elevated ketones in blood and urine, dehydration, and electrolyte imbalance. (See *ketoacidosis.*)

diabetic ketosis A serious state of diabetes in which there is glucose in blood and urine, ketones in blood and urine, and possibly some dehydration. (See *ketosis*).

dialysis A method of washing the toxins out of the blood. Peritoneal dialysis is done at home (usually four hours in, four hours out); hemodialysis is done at home (usually twelve hours in, twelve hours out) or at a center.

double-void technique The procedure of collecting a urine specimen thirty minutes after first voiding of all the urine. The double-voiding technique is often used in collecting urine to test for glucose and acetone levels. It is a rough measure of diabetes control at that particular time.

epinephrine A hormone released from the adrenal glands. Its main function in diabetes is to release glucose from the liver, increase the circulation rate, and prevent release of secreted insulin.

exchange A serving of food that contains known and relatively constant amounts of carbohydrate, fat, and/or protein. The food used in an exchange is usually weighed or measured. The exchanges are divided into several groups: milk, fruit, meat, fat, bread, and vegetables.

fasting blood glucose Blood-glucose concentration in the morning before breakfast. Commonly called fasting blood sugar (FBS).

fat One of the three main constituents of foods. Fats occur in nearly pure form as liquids or solids, such as oils and margarines, or they may be a component of other foods. Fats may be of animal or vegetable origin. They have a higher energy content than any other food (9 calories per gram).

fatty acids Constituents of fat. When there is an insulin deficiency, as in diabetes, fatty acids increase in the blood and are used by the liver to produce ketones.

flocculation A "snowy" look to insulin that may occur when the insulin has been exposed to too high or too low a temperature or when it is out of date.

fluorescein angiopathy Procedure in which photographs of the retina are taken after a water-soluble dye has been injected into the vein.

fractional urine Urine collected over a period of time and used to test for glucose and acetone levels. Fractions of urine are usually collected over twenty-four hours: from breakfast to lunchtime, from lunchtime to suppertime, from suppertime to bedtime, and from bedtime to rising. Also called block urine.

gangrene The death of tissue caused by a very poor blood supply, as sometimes occurs in the feet and legs of persons with diabetes. Infection may be a contributing cause.

genes Basic units of hereditary characteristics passed through reproduction (part of chromosomes).

gestational diabetes A period of abnormal glucose tolerance that occurs during pregnancy, usually controlled by diet and possibly insulin.

globin insulin Modified form of insulin produced by attaching a globin molecule to Regular insulin, slowing absorption and extending the peak and duration of action. Globin insulin is a clear insulin with acidic pH and intermediate action. It is no longer on the market.

glucagon A hormone produced by the alpha cells in the islet of Langerhans of the pancreas. Glucagon causes a rise in the blood-glucose level by releasing glucose from liver and muscle cells. It is used by injection for the treatment of severe insulin reactions at home, school, or work.

glucocorticoids Hormones released from the cortex of the adrenal gland; in relation to diabetes, they cause amino acids to be changed into new glucose (gluconeogenesis).

gluconeogenesis The process of converting amino acids and glycerol to new glucose. This process takes place in the liver and muscle cells of the body.

glucose The simple sugar, also known as dextrose, that is found in the blood and is used by the body for energy.

glucose tolerance The ability of the body to use and store glucose. Glucose tolerance is zero in persons with diabetes mellitus.

glucose-tolerance test A test for diabetes mellitus. The person being tested is given a measured amount of glucose to drink; blood-glucose levels are measured before ingestion and ½, 1½, 2, 3, and sometimes 4 to 6 hours after ingestion. Also called oral glucose tolerance test (OGTT).

glucose toxicity A state in which the lack of insulin, due to a decreased availability and/or function of the cell receptor site to receive insulin, results in an increase of glucose in the body, which is toxic to the beta cells in the islet of Langerhans. This toxicity is such that it may even lead to beta cell death.

glycogen Glycogen is glucose in storage form in the liver. It may be broken down to form blood glucose during an insulin reaction or during a fast.

glycogenesis The process whereby the liver converts a portion of glucose to glycogen.

glycogenolysis The breakdown of glycogen to glucose.

glycolysis The breakdown of glucose to carbon dioxide and water.

glycosuria The presence of glucose in the urine (*glyco* refers to sugar, *uria* to urine).

gram A small unit of weight in the metric system. Used in weighing food to determine a specific amount to eat or to burn in calories (1 pound [16 ounces] equals 453 grams).

heredity The transmission of a trait, such as blue eyes, from parents to offspring.

hormone A chemical substance produced by one gland or tissue and carried by the blood to other tissues or organs, where it stimulates action and causes a specific effect. Insulin and glucagon are hormones.

hyperbilirubinemia Condition in which a person has greater-than-normal value (+12.50 mg/dl in the infant) of bilirubin in the blood. Signs: jaundiced look to skin and whites of eyes.

hyperglycemia A greater-than-normal level of glucose in the blood (high blood glucose). Fasting blood-glucose values greater than 105 mg/dl (5.8 mMol) are suspect; greater than 140 mg/dl (7.8 mMol) are diagnostic.

hyperinsulinism An excessive amount of insulin, which may be caused by overpro-duction of insulin by the beta cells of the islets of Langerhans in the pancreas or by an excessive dose of insulin. Hyperinsulinism may cause hypoglycemia (low blood-glucose levels).

hypertension High blood pressure. Found to aggravate diabetes control or the complications already developed.

hypocalcemia Less-than-normal value (10–12 mg/dl in the infant) of calcium in the blood. Signs: convulsive seizure and irritability of the neuromuscular system.

hypoglycemia A less-than-normal level of glucose in the blood (low blood-glucose level). Fasting blood-glucose value less than 60 mg/dl (3.3 mMol).

hypoglycemic agent A drug or substance, such as sulfonylureas (e.g., Tolbutamide) and glipizide, used to reduce blood-glucose levels.

impaired glucose tolerance Condition that exists when blood-glucose values are elevated above normal but are inconclusive for diabetes. Sometimes mistakenly called borderline diabetes.

insulin A hormone secreted by the beta cells of the islets of Langerhans in the pancreas. Promotes the utilization of glucose.

insulin-dependent diabetes mellitus (IDDM) Also called

Type I diabetes or juvenile diabetes.

insulin reaction A condition with rapidly occurring onset that is the result of low blood-glucose levels. It may be caused by too much insulin, too little food, or an increase in exercise without a corresponding increase in food or decrease in insulin. Symptoms may vary from nervousness, shakiness, headaches, and drowsiness to confusion and convulsions, and even to coma.

intensive control Three or more doses of insulin per day or use of the insulin infusion pump with blood sugars in the normal or near normal range 80% or more of the time.

islets of Langerhans The small groups of cells in the pancreas that contain alpha, beta, and delta cells and produce glucagon, insulin, and somatostatin.

isophane insulin NPH (neutral protamine Hagedorn) insulin, a neutral pH, intermediate-acting insulin.

juvenile diabetes Now called *Type I* or *insulin-dependent diabetes mellitus* (IDDM).

ketoacidosis A condition of the body in which there is not enough insulin. Free fatty acids are released from fat cells and produce ketones in the liver. These ketones or acids result in an imbalance of the blood (acidosis). In the more acute state, the result is ketoacidosis. Large amounts of sugar and ketones are found in urine, electrolytes are imbalanced, and dehydration is present. The onset is usually slow. The condition leads to loss of appetite, abdominal pain, nausea and vomiting, rapid and deep respiration, and coma. Death may occur.

ketone bodies A name given by some to a mixture of ketones and other metabolism products that may break down into ketones. These other metabolism products are usually acetoacetic acid (which has a ketone group within the molecule) and beta hydroxybutyric acid (a molecule very similar to acetoacetic acid).

ketonemia The presence of ketones in the blood.

ketones Substances formed in the blood when a fat is broken down because of insufficient insulin. Fats are broken down into fatty acids, which are then chemically changed into ketones. Ketones (usually acetone) are often found in the blood and urine of persons with uncontrolled diabetes. Ketones may produce a fruity odor in the breath and urine of a person.

ketonuria The presence of ketones in the urine.

ketosis The presence of large amounts of ketones in the body, secondary to excessive breakdown of fat caused by insufficient insulin in a person with diabetes mellitus. Acidosis precedes and causes ketosis; the combination (ketosis and acidosis) is called ketoacidosis. Ketosis can also result from starvation or illness in nondiabetic individuals.

kidney threshold The level of a substance (such as glucose) in the blood in the kidney, above which it will be spilled into the urine. Also called renal threshold.

Kimmelstiel-Wilson syndrome Lesions of the filtered tubules of the kidney, caused by blood-vessel degeneration related to poorly controlled diabetes, as described by doctors Kimmelstiel and Wilson.

Kussmaul's respiration The rapid, deep, and labored respiration observed in patients with diabetic ketoacidosis; an involuntary mechanism to excrete carbon dioxide in order to reduce carbonic-acid level.

labile diabetes A term used for unstable diabetes control. (See *brittle diabetes*.)

Lente insulin An intermediate-acting insulin that is a mixture of 30 percent Semilente and 70 percent Ultralente insulin.

lipolysis The increased fat breakdown in the body tissues that occurs in ketosis (lysis of fat).

Liver Activation Treatment (Pulsatile IntraVenous Insulin Treatment) insulin given by vein in a pulse-like fashion (insulin based on total body needs given in short spurts every few seconds while the person sips a high glucose loaded drink).

macroangiopathy Disease related to the large blood vessels of the body.

maturity-onset diabetes Another name for Type II diabetes (also called adult diabetes, non–insulin-dependent diabetes, mild diabetes, ketone-resistant diabetes).

Mauriac syndrome A condition observed before puberty in children with prolonged, poorly controlled diabetes. It involves an enlarged, fatty liver, pitting edema, and short stature. The Mauriac syndrome is seldom seen today due to proper treatment, with adequate food and insulin provided for growth.

meal plan An arrangement whereby the total food allowed daily is expressed in terms of a certain number of points or exchanges, with the foods to be eaten at specific times.

metabolism All the chemical processes in the body, including those by which foods are broken down and used for tissue or energy production.

microaneurysms Small ballooned-out areas on the capillary blood vessels, such as might be found on the retina of the eye. They may burst and bleed.

microangiopathy Disease related to the small blood vessels of the body.

monounsaturated fat Has effect similar to that of polyunsaturated fat, but does not lower HDL cholesterol. Found in olive oil and other oils.

nephropathy Disease of the kidneys.

neuritis Inflammation of the nerves.

neuropathy Any disease of the nervous system. Neuropathy may occur in persons with diabetes and be related to poor control. Symptoms such as pain, loss of sensation, loss of reflexes, and/or weakness may occur.

non–insulin-dependent diabetes (NIDDM) Also called Type II diabetes.

NPH Neutral protamine Hagedorn, an intermediate-acting insulin that initially received its slower action through the addition of a protein to short-acting insulin.

omega Three fatty acids that are useful in lowering triglycerides and cholesterol. They also slow blood clotting. Found in salmon, tuna, and certain other fish.

open-loop system A mechanical system of insulin injection that is not self-controlled but must be controlled or programmed externally.

oral glucose-tolerance test (OGGT) See *glucose-tolerance test.*

oral hypoglycemia agent Another name for a blood-glucose-lowering agent. (See *hypoglycemic agent*).

pancreas A gland that is positioned near the stomach and that secretes at least two hormones—insulin and glucagon—and many digestive enzymes.

pancreas, artificial A mechanical device that stimulates the functions of the beta cells. It withdraws blood continuously, measures the glucose level, and injects an appropriate dose of insulin or glucose to reestablish a normal blood-glucose level.

points system A method of quantitating food intake by assigning points to various food components (carbohydrate, fat, protein, calories, sodium, etc.) and determining the number of each component point needed for a meal or for a day's intake. This system may either substitute for or accompany the less precise exchange system for diet calculation (75k = 1 point).

polydipsia Excessive thirst, with increased drinking of water.

polyphagia Excessive hunger or appetite, resulting in increased food intake.

polyunsaturated fat The type of fat that is liquid at room temperature, unless hydrogenated. Includes corn and certain other vegetable oils.

polyuria Excessive output of urine.

postprandial Occurring after a meal.

potential abnormality of glucose tolerance The time during the life of a diabetic person before any abnormality in glucose tolerance can be demonstrated. The identical twin of a person with diabetes is thought to have potential abnormality of glucose tolerance.

precipitate Particles that settle out of solution. This may occur in insulin that is kept beyond the expiration date, is contaminated, or is improperly mixed.

previous abnormality of glucose tolerance A classification used for the person who has been documented to have hyperglycemia during pregnancy, illness, or other crisis, but who currently has relatively normal blood-glucose levels without any treatment.

protamine zinc insulin (PZI) A long-acting insulin, prepared with large amounts of protamine combined with Regular insulin in the presence of zinc.

protein One of the three main constituents of foods. Proteins are made up of amino acids and are found in foods such as milk, meat, fish, and eggs. Proteins are essential constituents of all living cells and are the nitrogen-containing nutrient. The calorie content of protein is four calories per gram.

Regular insulin Short-acting insulin crystallized from the pancreas of animals or synthetically made. This insulin is neutralized and can be premixed with NPH insulin. Also known as clear insulin or crystalline insulin.

renal Pertaining to the kidneys.

renal threshold Another name for kidney threshold.

respiratory distress syndrome (RDS) Difficulty in breathing, noted by grunting, respiratory or expiratory wheezing or both, labored respiration, cyanosis (a blueness of the lips, face, fingers, and toes that can expand to involve the total body), and abnormal rate of respiration.

retina The light-sensitive layer at the back of the inner surface of the eyeball.

retinopathy Disease of the retina. Retinopathy occurs in persons with prolonged, poorly controlled diabetes and involves abnormal growth of and bleeding from the capillary blood vessels in the eye.

saturated fat The type of fat, such as butter, that is usually solid at room temperature. Saturated fats are usually derived from animal sources.

self-monitoring of blood glucose (SMBG) A technique of testing a person's blood-glucose level in order to determine the body response to activity, food, and medication.

Semilente Insulin prepared through special crystallizing techniques to produce small insulin crystals with large absorptive surfaces and rapid action. Semilente is slower in action than Regular insulin but more rapid than the intermediate-acting insulin.

serum glucose The concentration of glucose in the liquid part of the blood after the cells have been removed (clotted blood).

single-void technique The procedure of collecting a urine specimen four times a day, before meals and at bedtime. The bladder is not emptied for thirty minutes before the specimen is collected.

Somogyi effect A phenomenon (described by the biochemist Somogyi) in which hypoglycemia causes activation of the internal counterregulatory hormones (for example, glucagon, growth hormone, and epinephrine), causing a rebound in the blood-glucose level to hyperglycemic levels. Also called post-hypoglycemia hyperglycemia.

spot test A urine test performed on a sample collected using the single-void technique.

sulfonylureas Chemical compounds that stimulate production or release of insulin by the beta cells in the pancreas and/or prevent release of glucose from the liver. They are used in the treatment of Type II diabetes.

time-action curve A curve that shows the effect of a medicine at various times after it is taken.

twenty-four-hour urine Used to measure quantitative glucose levels in urine from a pooled, twenty-four-hour specimen.

Type I diabetes Results from inability to make insulin due to a combination of genetics or inheritance and environmental stressors. Insulin-dependent diabetes mellitus is associated with insulin's lack of availability, its action on the receptor sites, and/or its function with the glycolytic pathway. Also called insulin-dependent diabetes or juvenile diabetes.

Type II diabetes A type of diabetes that is usually found in adults over thirty years of age. The onset is gradual, and the symptoms are often minimal. Patients are often overweight. Those with Type II are less prone to acute complications, such as acidosis and coma, than are patients with Type I. Type II diabetes is treated through diet alone or through diet plus oral hypoglycemic agents. Insulin injections may or may not be required. Also called non–

insulin-dependent diabetes, non–ketosis-prone diabetes, or maturity-onset diabetes. (Previously called adult diabetes or maturity-onset diabetes in the young [MODY].)

Ultralente A long-acting insulin that is prepared using special crystallizing techniques that produce large crystals with small absorptive surfaces. Similar in action to PZI.

unsaturated fats The type of fat, such as vegetable oil, that is usually liquid at room temperature. (See *monounsaturated fat* and *polyunsaturated fat*.)

unstable diabetes Another name for *brittle diabetes*.

Bibliography

Chapter 1

Diabetes A to Z. 1988. Alexandria, Va.: American Diabetes Association.

The Diabetes Dictionary. 1989. Washington, D.C.: U.S. Dept. of Health and Human Services (National Diabetes Information Clearinghouse). NIH Pub. No. 89-3016.

What Is Non–Insulin-Dependent Diabetes (Type II Diabetes), and What Is Insulin-Dependent Diabetes (Type I Diabetes)? (pamphlet). 1989. Alexandria, Va.: American Diabetes Association.

Chapter 2

Diabetes: Facts You Need to Know. 1989. Alexandria, Va.: American Diabetes Association.

Direct and Indirect Costs of Diabetes. 1988. Alexandria, Va.: American Diabetes Association.

Miller, M. M., T. T. Gorski, and D. Miller. 1982. *Learning to Live Again.* Independence, Mo.: Independence Press.

Third-Party Reimbursement for Diabetes Outpatient Education: A Manual for Health-Care Professionals. 1986. Alexandria, Va.: American Diabetes Association.

Chapter 3

Balance Your Act: A Book for Adults with Diabetes. 1988. Atlanta, Ga.: Pritchett and Hull Associates, Inc.

Berstein, R. K. 1981. *Diabetes: the GlucoGraf Method for Normalizing Blood Sugar.* Los Angeles: J. P. Tarcher, Inc.

Biermann, J., and B. Toohey. 1988. *The Diabetic's Total Health Book.* Los Angeles: J. P. Tarcher, Inc.

Ducat, L., and S. Suib. 1983. *Diabetes: A New and Complete Guide to Healthier Living for Parents, Children, and Young Adults with Insulin-Dependent Diabetes Mellitus.* New York: Harper and Row.

Etzwiler, D., M. Franz, P. Hollander, and O. Joynes. 1987. *Learning to Live Well with Diabetes.* Wayzata, Minn.: Diabetes Center, Inc.

Managing Type II Diabetes: Your Invitation to a Healthier Lifestyle. 1988. Wayzata, Minn.: Diabetes Center, Inc.

Peterson, C. M., & L. Jovanovic. 1984. *The Diabetes Self-Care Method.* New York: Simon and Schuster.

Sims, D. G., ed. 1984. *Diabetes: Reach for Health and Freedom.* St. Louis, Mo.: C. V. Mosby.

Chapter 4

Curriculum for Youth Education. 1983. Alexandria, Va.: American Diabetes Association.

Diabetes: One Part of Me. 1988. Boston: Joslin Diabetes Center.

Diabetes Outpatient Education: The Evidence of Cost Savings. 1986. Alexandria, Va.: American Diabetes Association.

Guidelines for Education. 1988. Alexandria, Va.: American Diabetes Association.

Wheeler, M. 1989. "Choosing a Diabetes Education Program." *Diabetes Forecast,* Oct., 21–25.

Chapter 5

Barrett, A. 1984. *The Diabetic Brand-Name Food Exchange Handbook.* Philadelphia: Runing Press.

Calorie Points for Weight Control. 1987. Overland Park, Kans.: Nutrition Education Center.

Council on Scientific Affairs. "Treatment of Obesity in Adults." 1988. *Journal of the American Medical Association (JAMA)* 260(17): 2547–2551.

Exchange Lists for Meal Planning. 1986. Alexandria, Va.: American Diabetes Association.

Exchange Lists for Weight Management. 1989. Alexandria, Va.: American Diabetes Association.

Jovanovic, L., and C. M. Peterson, eds. 1985. *Nutrition and Diabetes.* New York: Alan R. Liss.

Nutrition for Children with Diabetes: A Pamphlet for Parents. 1987. Alexandria, Va.: American Diabetes Association.

Nutrition and Insulin-Dependent Diabetes (pamphlet). 1988. Alexandria, Va.: American Diabetes Association.

Nutrition and Non–Insulin-Dependent Diabetes (pamphlet). 1988. Alexandria, Va.: American Diabetes Association.

Palumbo, P. J., and J. D. Margie. 1987. *The Complete Diabetic Cookbook.* New York: New American Library.

Chapter 6

Bliss, M. *The Discovery of Insulin.* 1982. Chicago: University of Chicago Press.

Insulin. 1989. Ann Arbor, Mich.: University of Michigan.

Insulin Pump Therapy: Is It for You? 1986. Ann Arbor, Mich.: University of Michigan.

Oral Antidiabetes Medications. 1986. Ann Arbor, Mich.: University of Michigan.

Peragallo-Dittko, V. 1990. "Buyer's Guide to Injection Devices." *Diabetes Self-Management,* Jan.–Feb., 6–12.

Chapter 7

Armstrong, N., and D. Wakat. 1985. *The Energetic Diabetic: A Personal Fitness Guide.* Bowie, Md.: Brady Communications Company, Inc.

Biermann, J., and B. Toohey. 1977. *The Diabetic Sports and Exercise Book.* Philadelphia: Lippincott.

Diabetes and Exercise. 1988. Wayzata, Minn.: Diabetes Center, Inc.

Free to Be Fit: An Exercise Book for People with Type II Diabetes. 1989. Atlanta, Ga.: Pritchett and Hull Associates, Inc.

Ivy, J. 1990. "Exercise and Complications." *Diabetes Forecast,* 43(2): 46–49.

Wallace, J. P. 1989. "Exercise Myths." *Diabetes Forecast,* 42(6): 24–28.

Winter, J. 1984. *The Diabetic Get Fit Book.* New York: Arco Publishers.

Chapter 8

Diabetes and Impotence: A Concern for Couples. 1987. Wayzata, Minn.: Diabetes Center, Inc.

Diabetes Foot Care. 1986. Atlanta, Ga.: Pritchett and Hull Associates, Inc.

Periodontal Disease and Diabetes: A Guide for Patients. 1987. U.S. Department of Health and Human Services, NIH Pub. No. 87-2946.

Personal Health Habits for People with Diabetes. 1986. Ann Arbor, Mich.: University of Michigan.

Sexual Health and Diabetes. 1987. Ann Arbor, Mich.: University of Michigan.

Chapter 9

The Center for Diabetes Education. 1987. *Patterns: A Guidebook on How to Use Patterns in Glucose-Test Results in a Diabetes-Management Program.* Elkhart, Ind.: Miles, Inc.

Monitoring Your Diabetes. 1989. Ann Arbor, Mich.: University of Michigan.

Urine Testing for Ketones: Ketone Testing for the Person with Diabetes. 1987. Elkhart, Ind.: Miles, Inc.

Chapter 10

Caditz, J. 1989. *Diabetes, Visual Impairment, and Group Support: A Guidebook.* Santa Monica, Calif.: Center for the Partially Sighted.

Diabetic Retinopathy and Its Treatment by Laser. 1986. Ann Arbor, Mich.: University of Michigan.

Hyperglycemia, Hypoglycemia, and Various Other Complications Of Diabetes (pamphlet). 1988–

89. Alexandria, Va.: American Diabetes Association.

Jovanovic, L., J. Biermann, and B. Toohey. 1987. *The Diabetic Woman: All Your Questions Answered.* Los Angeles: J. P. Tarcher, Inc.

Long-Term Complications. 1988. Ann Arbor, Mich.: University of Michigan.

Special Report: DCCT: What it means to you. Alexandria, VA: American Diabetes Association, September 1993.

Chapter 11

Anderson, B., M. T. Burkhart, and D. Charron-Prochownik. 1986. *Making Choices: Teenagers and Diabetes.* Ann Arbor, Mich.: University of Michigan.

Biermann, J., and B. Toohey. 1984. *The Peripatetic Diabetic.* Los Angeles: J. P. Tarcher, Inc.

Bradley, D. J. 1987. *What Does It Feel Like to Have Diabetes? A Diary of Events in the Life of a Diabetic.* Springfield, Ill.: Charles C. Thomas.

Diabetes and You (A Pamphlet for Parents, Children, Teenagers, Young Adults, Adults, and Senior Adults). 1987–88. Alexandria, Va.: American Diabetes Assocation.

Edelwich, J., and A. Brodsky. 1986. *Diabetes: Caring for Your Emotions as Well as Your Health.* Reading, Mass.: Addison-Wesley.

Feste, C. 1987. *Physician Within: Taking Charge of Your Well-Being.* Wayzata, Minn.: Diabetes Center, Inc.

Kleiman, G., and S. Dody. 1986. *No Time to Lose.* New York: William Morrow.

Anderson, B., M. T. Burkhart, and D. Charron-Prochownik. 1986.

McLean, T. 1986. *Metal Jam—the Story of a Diabetic.* New York: St. Martin's Press.

Piotrowski, M., and Sochalski. 1986. *Learning to Live with Diabetes.* Ann Arbor, Mich.: University of Michigan.

Pray, L. M., and R. Evans. 1983. *Journey of a Diabetic.* New York: Simon and Schuster.

Register, C. 1987. *Living with Chronic Illness.* New York: The Free Press.

Rubin, R.R., Biermann, J., Toohey, B. 1992. *Psyching Out diabetes.* Los Angeles: Lowell House.

Shalom, R., and J. J. Ryan. 1989. *Diabetes Support Groups for Young Adults: A Facilitator's Manual.* Alexandria, Va.: American Diabetes Association.

Chapter 12

Cuban, B. 1989. "Getting the Best of Stress." *Diabetes Forecast,* 42(6): 42–45.

Eliot, R. S., and D. L. Breo. 1984. *Is It Worth Dying for a Self-Assessment Program to Make Stress Work for You, Not*

Against You? New York: Bantam Books.

Faelten, S., and D. Diamond. 1988. *Take Control of Your Life: A Complete Guide to Stress Relief.* Emmaus, Pa.: Rodale Press.

Hanson, P. G. 1986. *The Joy of Stress: How to Make Stress Work for You.* New York: Andrews, McMeel & Parker.

Krieger, D. 1979. *The Therapeutic Touch: How to Use Your Hands to Help or to Heal.* Englewood Cliffs, N.J.: Prentice-Hill.

"Taking the Confusion Out of Stress Advice." 1990. *Diabetes in the News,* 9(1): 9–21, 24.

Wolf, F. M., L. S. Robins, et al. 1985. *Exercising for Relaxation and Fitness: The Easy-Does-It Program with Special Tips for People with Diabetes and Heart Disease.* Ann Arbor, Mich.: University of Michigan.

Chapter 13

Lodewick, P. A. 1987. *A Diabetic Doctor Looks at Diabetes—His and Yours.* Cambridge, Mass.: RMI Corporation.

Chapter 15

"American Diabetes Association Research Report." 1990. *Diabetes Forecast,* 43(3): 37–52.

Juvenile Diabetes Foundation. 1990. "The Rising Costs of Diabetes Research." *Countdown,* Spring, 7–11.

Index

241

Diagnosis of diabetes, reaction to,
111–112
Diet, diabetic, 31–32. *See also* Food(s);
Meal planning; Nutrition
Down's syndrome, 10
Drugs. *See* Medications, for diabetes
Dymelor. *See* Acetohexamide

Eating. *See* Diet, diabetic; Food(s);
Meal planning; Nutrition;
Restaurants
Education about diabetes, 1, 25–30
after diagnosis, 111–112
for family members, 18, 29,
130–131, 133
home-management level, 26–27
programs available for, 28–29
self-management level, 5, 27–28
survival level, 25–26
value of, 29–30
Egyptians, 3
Emotional response to diabetes.
See Grief response; Stress,
emotional
Endorphins, 120
Exchange lists, 36, 158–174
combination foods, 170–171
defined, 157
fat list, 168–169
free foods, 169–170
fruit list, 165–167
meat list, 161–164
milk list, 167–168
starch/bread list, 159–161
vegetable list, 165
Exercise, 63–70
aerobic, 63, 64
anaerobic, 66
benefits of, 63–66
and blood-glucose level, 66
and eating, 67–68
and hypoglycemia, 69
with partner, 68
precautions, 66, 68–69
recommendations for, 69–70
and sensitivity of cell receptor sites
to insulin, 64
target rate heart zone, 64–65
value of, 123
warning signs, *68*
Eye care, 77–78
Eye problems. *See* Retinopathy

Family members, 111–112, 130–133
education about diabetes, 18, 29,
130–131, 133
meetings, 132
support of, 115–116
Fats, dietary, 32, 33–34. *See also*
Cholesterol; Triglycerides
types of, *33*
Feet. *See* Foot care; Foot problems
Food(s), 4. *See also* Meal planning
absorption of, 31
calorie-points, 178–180
exchange lists, 158–174
and exercise, 66, 68
managing diabetes with, 154–155
for preventing hypoglycemia, 39
questionnaire, 144–147
for treating hypoglycemia, 101
Food points system, 36. *See also*
Calorie-points
Foot care, 74–77, 106
steps in, *74*
Foot problems, 75
Friends, 111–112, 130–133
educating about diabetes, 130–131,
133
Fructosamine test, 84, 85, 95
Funding for research, 142–143

General Adaptation Syndrome,
119–120
Genetic markers, 138
Gestational diabetes, 9–10, 23
Gingivitis, 71, 72
Glipizide, *42*, 44–45
Glossaries of diabetes-related terms,
175–177, 224–235
Glucagon, 4, 101, *102*
Glucose, storage of food as, 32
Glucose levels. *See* Blood-glucose
levels; Blood-glucose testing
Glucose testing strips, 88
Glucose tolerance, impaired, 8–9
Glucosuria, *98*
Glucotrol. *See* Glipizide
Glyburide, *42*, 44
Glycosylated hemoglobin test, 95
and blood-glucose levels, 84–85
information provided by, 80
problems with, 84
testing, 81
Grief response, 112–113